Attachment-Based Family Therapy

for Sexual and Gender Minority Young Adults
and Their Nonaccepting Parents

Diamond and Boruchovitz-Zamir have developed the only evidence-based psycho-therapy to help LGBTQ people and their parents resolve the often-unacknowledged, painful tensions that can linger between them. Every page of this book shines with clinical wisdom, concrete guidance, and compassion derived from the authors' many years of firsthand experience working with these families. Therapists will do a tremendous service to LGBTQ people and their families by reading this book and applying its intuitive, accessible lessons to their own practice.

—**John Pachankis, PhD,** Susan Dwight Bliss Professor of Public Health, Yale University, New Haven, CT, United States

This is the definitive work on this new and effective treatment for families struggling to stay connected. Attachment-based family therapy is a theoretically grounded, highly teachable treatment, and this rich description of it is rendered with clarity and empathy. Highly recommended!

—**Laurie Heatherington, PhD,** Edward Dorr Griffin Professor of Psychology Emerita, Williams College, Williamstown, MA, United States

The authors describe a step-by-step process for conducting attachment-based family therapy for sexual and gender minority young adults and their nonaccepting parents. The ideas presented are very clear, and the book is well-structured, integrated, and organized. This excellent book will make a fantastic addition to the literature for family therapists and especially those who work with families of LGBTQ+ adolescents and young adults.

—**Yochay Nadan, PhD,** Associate Professor, The Hebrew University of Jerusalem, Jerusalem, Israel; Social Worker; and Licensed Couple and Family Therapist and Supervisor

Diamond and Boruchovitz-Zamir's book is a hands-on clinical guide that walks therapists through the theory, structure, and mechanics of attachment-based family therapy for sexual and gender minority young adults and their nonaccepting parents. For the purposes of growth and transformation, the authors provide a clear strategy for helping families attune to the pain of feeling disconnected from one another as well as the incredible strength that comes from relationship repair. Through illustrative case examples and narratives, the authors take us into the room with their client families, help us to experience therapeutic emotional shifts, and allow us to witness the rebuilding of "sacred trust" through their work. Most important, we are reminded that parents are willing to come into contact with difficult emotions, such as pain and fear, for the sake of their young adult and can, therefore, use their caregiving instinct to respond in ways that have been previously unavailable to them. A powerful prompt for therapists to harness the attachment capabilities of parents in therapeutic practice with LGBTQ+ young adults.

—**Jody Russon, PhD, LMFT,** Department of Human Development and Family Science, Virginia Tech, Blacksburg, VA, United States

Attachment-Based Family Therapy

for Sexual and Gender Minority Young Adults and Their Nonaccepting Parents

Gary M. Diamond
Rotem Boruchovitz-Zamir

 AMERICAN PSYCHOLOGICAL ASSOCIATION

Published by
American Psychological Association
750 First Street, NE
Washington, DC 20002
https://www.apa.org

Order Department
https://www.apa.org/pubs/books
order@apa.org

In the U.K., Europe, Africa, and the Middle East, copies may be ordered from Eurospan
https://www.eurospanbookstore.com/apa
info@eurospangroup.com

Typeset in Charter and Interstate by Circle Graphics, Inc., Reisterstown, MD

Printer: Gasch Printing, Odenton, MD
Cover Designer: Anthony Paular Design, Newbury Park, CA

Library of Congress Cataloging-in-Publication Data

Names: Diamond, Gary M., author. | Boruchovitz-Zamir, Rotem, author. |
   American Psychological Association, issuing body.
Title: Attachment-based family therapy for sexual and gender minority young
   adults and their nonaccepting parents / by Gary M. Diamond and Rotem
   Boruchovitz-Zamir.
Description: Washington, DC : American Psychological Association, [2023] |
   Includes bibliographical references and index.
Identifiers: LCCN 2022045765 (print) | LCCN 2022045766 (ebook) |
   ISBN 9781433836619 (paperback) | ISBN 9781433840913 (ebook)
Subjects: MESH: Object Attachment | Family Therapy--methods | Sexual and
   Gender Minorities--psychology | Parent-Child Relations | Young Adult |
   BISAC: PSYCHOLOGY / Psychotherapy / LGBTQ | FAMILY & RELATIONSHIPS /
   LGBTQ
Classification: LCC RC488.5 (print) | LCC RC488.5 (ebook) | NLM WM
   460.5.O2 | DDC 616.89/156--dc23/eng/20221115
LC record available at https://lccn.loc.gov/2022045765
LC ebook record available at https://lccn.loc.gov/2022045766

https://doi.org/10.1037/0000352-000

Printed in the United States of America

10 9 8 7 6 5 4 3 2 1

Contents

Preface

The birth of attachment-based family therapy for sexual and gender minority young adults and their nonaccepting parents (ABFT-SGM) can be traced back to 2005, the year I (GMD) took a 2-year sabbatical from my position as a professor of psychology at Ben-Gurion University in Israel to go to Philadelphia to serve as the codirector of the Center for Family Intervention Science at the Children's Hospital of Philadelphia. I had been invited by Guy S. Diamond (no family relation), director of the center, primary developer of attachment-based family therapy (ABFT) for depressed and suicidal adolescents, close colleague, and dear friend.

At the time, Guy and I had already been working together for 8 years. He had supervised me from 1996 to 1998 as a predoctoral intern and then as a postdoctoral clinical psychology fellow at the Philadelphia Child Guidance Clinic. I had served as a therapist in his first randomized clinical trial of ABFT for depressed adolescents, and we had spent hours and hours talking about cases and refining the treatment model. Even after I returned to Israel in 1998, we continued our collaboration. My lab members and I have conducted numerous studies on the purported change processes underlying ABFT, including the therapeutic alliance, therapist adherence, the immediate effect of relational reframes and other therapist interventions, emotional processing, and corrective attachment episodes.

When I returned to Philadelphia in 2005, Guy and his team were already in the midst of a second randomized clinical trial, comparing ABFT to enhanced usual care for suicidal adolescents. Suzanne Levy had joined the team and has since become a codeveloper of the ABFT model, master therapist and supervisor, director of training, and friend. In my role as codirector at the time, I supervised many of the study cases in this second clinical trial. What quickly became apparent was that a substantial number of the adolescents we were seeing were openly identifying as lesbian, gay, bisexual, transgender, and queer (LGBTQ+; see Chapter 1 for a discussion of our choice of terminology). Sometimes their parents' nonacceptance of their identity was a driving force behind their suicidal ideation. Sometimes it was not. In either case, it was clear that we, as a team, had not yet sufficiently considered the unique experiences of sexual and gender minority adolescents and their families or how to ensure that ABFT was sensitive to, and would meet, these families' needs.

In 2007, I received a grant from the American Foundation for Suicide Prevention to systematically adapt ABFT for sexual minority depressed and suicidal adolescents. Together with Suzanne and Guy, we put together a treatment development team, conducted focus groups with LGBTQ+ partners in the field, and adapted the model in important ways. We then conducted a pilot trial in which we treated 10 lesbian, gay, and bisexual suicidal and depressed adolescents and their parents. The results from this seminal project were encouraging (G. M. Diamond et al., 2012).

After returning to Israel in 2007, my doctoral student Maya Shpigel and I began working with LGBTQ+ young adults and their nonaccepting parents. These families turned to us not because the young adult was depressed or suicidal (although some were) but because they felt like their relationships had been diminished or even shattered since the young adult's coming out. Often the young adult longed to find a way to remain connected to their parents in a loving, safe, mutually accepting, and meaningful way while still living an authentic, full life. Parents, for their part, were searching for a way to work through their fear, shame, and sense of loss and be involved in their young adult's life in a more positive, consistent, and supportive manner.

In 2015, we received funding from the Israel Science Foundation to conduct the first open clinical trial of ABFT-SGM for young adults and their nonaccepting parents. We found that over the course of the treatment, parents became less rejecting and more accepting. We also found that young adults reported feeling increasingly more comfortable sharing their thoughts and feelings with their parents and going to them for support during moments of distress (G. M. Diamond et al., 2022). This book presents—for the first time—the complete manual for conducting ABFT-SGM.

In 2013, in a moment of synchronicity, my then 16-year-old son, Orian, came out to my wife, Rivi, and me. In many ways, it was not a big surprise to us. Orian had always displayed some gender atypical behaviors and interests. Rivi and I had periodically talked between ourselves about the possibility that he might be gay. We made sure to be explicit about our accepting, affirmative attitudes and to support and encourage his unique, amazing qualities and talents. What *was* a surprise for me was that, despite my attitudes, beliefs, awareness, and commitment to embracing and celebrating both of my sons for the unique special people that they are, at that moment, I suddenly felt a pit in my stomach. Rivi and I both hugged Orian long and hard and told him how much we loved him and were proud of him. There was never any doubt about our acceptance and support.

With Orian's permission, we immediately shared our news with extended families and friends. As we expected, they all responded in an affirming, supportive manner. Yet, I was left puzzled by that fleeting moment of distress. It felt visceral. It had bypassed my frontal cortex. Was it fear about how others might perceive Orian? Fear about the challenges I imagined he might face in life? Shame or fear about how I imagined others might perceive me and my family? Grief regarding the loss of my heteronormative dreams about our future family?

Over the ensuing years, Orian's journey—and our journey together—has inspired and taught me. It has enabled me to connect with the families we treat in a deeper, more personal way. It has informed the way I work. With that said, I am acutely aware that my family's experience is much different from that of many of the families that come to us for help. In many ways, we are extremely privileged. We are surrounded by open, accepting extended family, friends, and community. Orian is fortunate to live and work in a relatively safe, affirming environment. Also, he does not have the additional layers of stressors many people of color and transgender people face. This book is for therapists working with families that, for whatever reasons, have gotten stuck somewhere along the acceptance process and are looking for a way to move forward and deepen their bonds.

My (RBZ) part in ABFT-SGM started when I arrived at Gary's lab for the first time as a beginning graduate student. I had worked for several years with Nava Levit-Binnun and Yulia Golland as an undergraduate research assistant. Their work, studying the mechanisms of social interaction and connectedness, fascinated me. It inspired me to research the therapeutic effects that deep, loving relationships have on people's well-being. Meeting Gary and joining his lab was a true gift. It was everything I could hope for in my training as a researcher and therapist. I felt immediately connected to ABFT-SGM, to its relational focus and client-driven approach, and to its commitment to promoting the special and unique connection between parents and their children, even when family members themselves are struggling to believe.

Acknowledgments

Many people have contributed over the years to the work presented here. I (GMD) first and foremost thank Rotem (Boruchovitz-Zamir): colleague, codeveloper of attachment-based family therapy for sexual and gender minority young adults and their nonaccepting parents (ABFT-SGM), coauthor, and expert therapist. This book would not be what it is—or perhaps even exist—without you. To Guy (Diamond) and Suzanne (Levy): One could not hope for better colleagues and friends. Your ideas and clinical wisdom are reflected in every aspect of the model and throughout the book. Thank you for support.

I also thank Howard Liddle: supervisor, teacher, and mentor. Howard taught me how to think and work with subsystems as well as prepare for and conduct transformative in-session enactments. His passion for doing psychotherapy research ignited in me a flame that has moved me forward throughout my career. I thank, too, Jody Russon, who has taken the lead on developing attachment-based family therapy for gender minority depressed and suicidal adolescents, and who provided invaluable comments on this book manuscript.

I thank all of the graduate students and therapists who, over the years, have been an integral part of developing and testing ABFT-SGM. Thank you to Maya Shpigel, Nitzan Cohen, Dana Stolowitz, Yael Belsky, Rotem, Ofir Nir-Gottlieb, Inbal Gat, Maayan Dor, Priel-Yehoshua Fitoussi, Chen Lifshitz, Noa Tsvieli, Shira Katz, Tamar Zisenwine, Yotam Strifler, Ella Kibrik, Ayelet Levy, and Lisa Rozenblat. We could not have done it without you. Also, a special thanks to Susan L. Reynolds, acquisitions editor at the American Psychological Association (APA), who guided us through the writing of the book with the skill of a seasoned therapist. Thanks also to Krissy Jones, APA development editor, who took over for Susan after the manuscript was submitted and pushed us across the finish line.

I thank my loving family: my parents, Beverly and Stan; my sister, Jodi, and brother-in-law, Lenny; my dearest wife and best friend, Rivi; and my sons, Orian and Yahel. You are my rock, my biggest fans, and my most important teachers. To Orian and Yahel, who periodically pushed me forward by chanting, "Where's the book? Where's the book?" at Friday night dinners: "Here's the book!"

Finally, both Rotem and I thank the amazing, inspiring families who have courageously opened their hearts and souls to us and to each other. These families who have overcome their fears and let their love and commitment for one another lead them forward. Thank you for trusting us and letting us be a small part of your lives.

I (RBZ) express my gratitude to Gary (Diamond), for everything that you have taught me, for including me in the development of ABFT-SGM, and for inviting me to write this book with you. It has been a true honor and privilege. I also thank Ofir Nir-Gottlieb, Inbal Gat, and Ella Givon, my friends and fellow cotherapists. I owe a lot of what I know as a therapist to your wisdom and friendship.

A deep thanks goes to my beloved parents, Boro and Irit, and my sisters, Tamar and Yael. Thank you for being the loving, supportive family you are. It is no wonder I grew up to think family is such a crucial part of being whole.

Finally, I thank Arnon, my life partner and closest friend, and our incredible sons, Itamar and Uriya. The three of you are my home, my biggest pride, and my life's happiness.

Attachment-Based Family Therapy

for Sexual and Gender Minority Young Adults
and Their Nonaccepting Parents

1 INTRODUCTION TO ATTACHMENT-BASED FAMILY THERAPY FOR SEXUAL AND GENDER MINORITY YOUNG ADULTS AND THEIR NONACCEPTING PARENTS

Although homosexuality is still denounced or even criminalized in many parts of the world, Western society as a whole has become increasingly accepting of lesbian, gay, bisexual, transgender, and queer (LGBTQ+)[1] people. LGBTQ+ people are more visible in almost all spheres of public life. In many countries, important antidiscrimination laws have been passed, and same-sex marriages are now recognized. That said, individual attitudes remain deeply divided. More than a quarter of Americans still view same-sex orientation as unacceptable. Moreover, increased societal acceptance and legal protections for LGBTQ+ people have sparked a dramatic backlash. For example, the United States is currently seeing a surge in anti-LGBTQ+ rhetoric and policies, including an extraordinary legal assault on transgender rights and the rights of parents to provide their trans children with gender-affirming medical care. Florida recently passed a law banning any discussions about sexual orientation and gender in kindergarten through third grade. Shortly thereafter, a member of

[1]We use the terms *LGBTQ+* and *sexual and gender minority* interchangeably throughout this book to refer to the full range of people who are stigmatized because of whom they are attracted to, their sexual behavior or gender expression, or their self-identification. We discuss our choice of terminology later in this chapter.

https://doi.org/10.1037/0000352-001

Attachment-Based Family Therapy for Sexual and Gender Minority Young Adults and Their Nonaccepting Parents, by G. M. Diamond and R. Boruchovitz-Zamir

the U.S. Supreme Court suggested that federal laws protecting LGBTQ+ rights, including the right to marry, should be reconsidered. Such nonaccepting, reactionary views are more prevalent in conservative communities and are often grounded in religious fundamentalism, identity politics, and a fear of change and otherness (Drumheller & McQuay, 2010; Rosenkrantz et al., 2020; van der Toorn et al., 2017).

Perhaps nowhere are attitudes more evenly divided than in Israel, where we (GMD and RBZ) live and work. The most recent Pew Research Center survey found that whereas half of Israelis accept homosexuality, the other half does not. Moreover, these figures have not changed over the past decade (Poushter & Kent, 2020). Although the predominantly liberal and secular metropolis of Tel Aviv has consistently been voted one of the world's most gay-friendly cities, same-sex couples still cannot marry in Israel. On the one hand, 5% of Israeli parliament members are openly gay—the fourth highest percentage in the world—yet, on the other hand, leading rabbis, educators, and politicians continue to openly and unabashedly spread hateful, homophobic, and transphobic messages. During the 2015 Gay Pride parade in Jerusalem, an ultraorthodox Jew stabbed to death a 16-year-old marching in support of LGBTQ+ rights (PBS News Weekend, 2015). In 2022, the Pride parade scheduled for June in the southern Israeli town of Netivot was canceled after a bullet was left at the office door of the mother of a parade organizer (*The Times of Israel* Staff, 2022). Indeed, the most recent (2020) findings from The Aguda, The Association for LGBTQ Equality in Israel, showed that hate speech and violent acts against LGBTQ+ individuals in Israel rose by 27% in just 1 year alone, with transgender people being particularly targeted (Dvir, 2021).

As Stone Fish and Harvey (2005) pointed out, it is impossible to grow up in a culture in which heterosexist, homophobic, and transphobic messages are prevalent and not be affected by such messages. It is no wonder that most parents experience some degree of fear, shame, and loss on learning that their own child is same-sex oriented or gender nonconforming. Some parents perceive being LGBTQ+ as unnatural, a flaw, a liability. They worry about how others, including their friends and extended family members, will react. They are afraid that they will be pitied, ridiculed, or judged and that people will distance themselves from them. They grieve the loss of their hetero- and gender-normative dream of sitting around the dinner table with their child, his or her opposite-sex spouse, and biological grandchildren. They are forced to let go of the future they once imagined. Some parents panic about their child's welfare, afraid that they will be taken advantage of, discriminated against, and victimized. They imagine a dark future in which their child is living alone, marginalized, miserable, and unfulfilled, with no support system or joy in their life. Those parents who are religious may face the additional challenge of reconciling their love for their child with their beliefs that homosexuality is immoral. They may be afraid that those in their religious community will judge or shun them and their child.

Parents' fear, shame, sense of loss, and anger can lead them to reject their young adult's[2] sexual or gender identity. Such parental rejection can manifest in many different ways. In extreme cases, parents may humiliate their young adult (e.g., "Stop acting like a woman") or invalidate their lived experience (e.g., "I know what and who you are better than you know yourself, and you are not a lesbian"). Some may attempt to coerce their young adult into trying to "change" their orientation, gender identity, or behavior (e.g., "I'm not willing to help support you if you choose to live with a woman"). Less direct, but still painful, forms of parental rejection include withdrawing from their young adult. Parents may spend less time with their young adult, be less emotionally involved in their lives, and be less physically affectionate with them. They may also ask their young adult to conceal their identity from certain family members or acquaintances (e.g., "I don't want Mum-mum to know").

Sometimes parents convey their lack of acceptance via more subtle messages. For example, one genderqueer young adult we (GMD, RBZ, and colleagues) worked with described how hurt and invalidated she feels each time her mother raises her eyebrows in a sign of disapproval when noticing that she is wearing nail polish. Such subtle, negative, invalidating messages directed toward stigmatized or marginalized people, including LGBTQ+ individuals, have been termed *microaggressions* (Balsam et al., 2011; Sue, 2010). Although most parents become more accepting, or at least more tolerant, over time, others remain partially or fully rejecting, even years after learning of their child's identity (Beals & Peplau, 2006; Cramer & Roach, 1988; Grossman et al., 2021; Samarova et al., 2014).

Ongoing parental criticism, invalidation, and rejection of one's sexual or gender identity can take a profound psychological toll. Such criticism, invalidation, and rejection are associated with young adults' internalized

---

[2]We have chosen the term *young adult* as opposed to "youth," "emerging adults," or "adults" because most of the young adults we work with are between 25 and 40 years old. This age range is thought to represent a unique development stage, distinguishable from emerging adulthood on the one hand and adulthood on the other (Arnett, 2000). That said, we have found this work appropriate for emerging adults, ages 20 to 25 who are no longer living in their home, and for adult children older than 40.

homophobia, expectations for future gay-related rejection by others (Pachankis et al., 2008), depression, suicidal ideation, anxiety symptoms (D'Augelli et al., 2005; Kibrik et al., 2019; Remafedi et al., 1991; Ryan et al., 2009), and drug and alcohol consumption (D'Amico & Julien, 2012; Padilla et al., 2010; Rothman et al., 2012).

Parental rejection can also destroy the fabric of family relationships. Young adults may distance themselves from their parents to protect themselves from being hurt and frustrated. They may avoid family events, particularly when parents are unwilling to include their partner or refuse to address them using their preferred names or pronouns. Even when spending time together, conversations may be constricted and shallow or emotionally loaded and quick to escalate. Both parents and their young adult may feel like they are walking on eggshells. Over the course of time, such dynamics erode relationships. Relationships become superficial, strained, conflicted, detached or cut off. Family members feel increasingly hopeless, resentful, and alone. What may have once felt like loving, secure, meaningful, and nurturing family bonds—a secure base and safe haven that could always be counted on—now feels fragile, tenuous, toxic or nonexistent.

In contrast, when parents are accepting of their young adult's sexual or gender minority identity, it has a positive effect on the self of the young adult and on the young adult–parent relationship (Ryan et al., 2009, 2010). Importantly, such acceptance is not simply the absence of rejection but rather overt supportive and affirming behaviors that convey to the young adult that they are prized and admired for who they are (D'Amico & Julien, 2012; Kibrik et al., 2019; Ryan et al., 2010). Parental acceptance means actively encouraging one's young adult to be themselves. Accepting parents are proud of their children and affirm their identity. They show interest in their young adult's personal life. They make an effort to both get to know their young adult's friends and partners and to include them in family events. Accepting parents come out to family and friends, stand up for their child, and advocate for their child's rights.

Not surprisingly, parental acceptance is associated with young adults' lower rates of suicidal thoughts and suicide attempts, higher levels of perceived social support, lower levels of psychological symptoms, and better general health (Kibrik et al., 2019; Ryan et al., 2010). When young adults feel accepted by their parents, they feel better about themselves (Ryan et al., 2010). They internalize their parents' interest, care, and pride in them. This positive view of the self helps the young adult to feel confident, explore, take chances, allow themselves to be vulnerable, and remain resilient in the face of negative life events. Indeed, self-esteem has been linked to well-being, goal attainment, and better interpersonal relationships (Harris & Orth, 2020).

Parental acceptance also allows sexual and gender minority young adults to remain positively connected to their parents. Research findings show that emerging and young adults in general, unrelated to sexual orientation or gender identity, report that their parents are one of their most important relationships and a primary source of support (Arnett, 2014; Fingerman et al., 2012). When parents accept their young adult's identity and autonomy, while at the same time provide support and closeness, young adults feel worthwhile, secure, and connected (Aquilino, 2006). Their bond with their parents is integral to young adults' well-being and functioning in the world and is on par with their relationships with romantic partners and peers (van Wel et al., 2000, 2002).

For sexual and gender minority young adults, such parental support and connection may be even more critical because they are subjected to minority stress. *Minority stress* refers to the stress LGBTQ+ people experience as a consequence of being marginalized, discriminated against, and victimized because of their stigmatized identity. It also refers to the stress associated with understandable yet maladaptive responses to such prejudice and victimization, including internalized homophobia, identity concealment, and rejection sensitivity (Hatzenbuehler et al., 2009; Meyer, 2003). When LGBTQ+ young adults can turn to and use their parents for support when facing such stressors, and parents are available to help their young adult process their emotions, problem solve, and feel less alone, it serves to buffer against the negative effects of minority stress. Indeed, research has shown that parental support moderates the negative effects of gay-related victimization (Evans et al., 2004; Shilo et al., 2015) and the association between minority sexual orientation and suicidal thoughts (Eisenberg & Resnick, 2006; Needham & Austin, 2010). Even when there is no immediate stressor, feeling connected to parents engenders a sense of safety and well-being. The young adult knows that whatever might happen, they are not alone (L. M. Diamond & Alley, 2022).

Whereas the idea of helping parents and their sexual and gender minority young adults form more accepting, open, closer relationships may have seemed almost inconceivable 50 years ago, times and attitudes are changing. Greater societal acceptance has created new possibilities and expectations. Positive role models of accepting families fill our television and movie screens. Most parents have a family member, friend, or colleague who is openly LGBTQ+. Many places of worship now advertise that they are LGBTQ+ friendly. All of this makes it possible for an increasing number of parents and their LGBTQ+ adult children to imagine being connected in an open, loving, and meaningful manner.

Therapists' expectations and goals for such families have also changed. In the past, treatment typically focused on helping LGBTQ+ young adults manage their parents' rejecting behaviors and move on with their lives. Parents were usually not involved in the therapy. Instead, the emphasis was on protecting the young adult from toxic family interactions; mourning the loss of their relationships with their biological parents; and identifying new, alternative sources of social support, such as "chosen" families. Today, however, therapists know that parents can change and that relationships between LGBTQ+ young adults and their parents can be transformed (G. M. Diamond et al., 2022). Therapists are more likely to work with families in an effort to facilitate greater acceptance; repair relational ruptures; and promote safe, mutually respectful and open relationships that allow family members to remain meaningfully connected. A number of excellent professional books have been written about how to help families navigate the coming out process, facilitate parental acceptance, and transform parent–child relationships (e.g., Harvey & Stone Fish, 2015; LaSala, 2010; Stone Fish & Harvey, 2005). Our (GMD and RBZ's) experience is that deep down, most sexual and gender minority young adults long to feel loved by, and remain positively connected to, their parents. Likewise, most parents long to feel good about their child, share in their joys, and be there to support them in tough times.

PURPOSE OF THIS BOOK

This book describes the step-by-step process of conducting attachment-based family therapy for sexual and gender minority young adults and their non-accepting parents (ABFT-SGM). ABFT-SGM for this population is specifically designed to help reduce parental rejection; facilitate parental acceptance; and, ultimately, promote safe, mutually respectful, closer, validating, loving, authentic, and meaningful relationships between LGBTQ+ young adults and their parents. The treatment is meant for families that continue to experience ongoing frustration, disappointment, conflict, grief, or distance in their relationships months or even years after their young adult has come out.

TERMINOLOGY

An abundance of terms has been used to describe people who are not exclusively heterosexual or cisgender (Eliason, 2014). Perhaps the most common and recognizable are the labels "lesbian," "gay," "bisexual," and "transgender."

Such labels, however, are limited. They do not always capture the person's lived experience or account for the full range and variety in sexual attraction, sexual behavior, gender identity, and gender performance. For example, the term "transgender," typically used to refer to a person whose gender identity differs from the sex that they were assigned at birth, may not align with the experience of a person who feels that their gender goes beyond simply identifying as either a man or a woman. Such people may feel that terms such as "nonbinary" or "genderqueer" better capture their identity. For others, labels in general may feel restrictive, irrelevant, or even offensive, and they may prefer not to label themselves. Such might be the case with two women in a committed romantic relationship who do not conceive of themselves as lesbian or bisexual. Most labels also do not capture the dynamic nature of sexuality and gender, which can fluctuate and evolve over time (L. M. Diamond, 2006).

In our clinical work, we (GMD and RBZ) ask the young adult what language or terms best suit them and then use that language in our work together. For the purposes of this book, however, we have chosen to use a single set of terms for the sake of clarity. We did so, recognizing that no single term or set of terms fully reflects the varied experiences of our clients. In the end, we chose to use the terms *sexual and gender minority* and *LGBTQ+* to refer to people whose same-sex orientation, attraction, or behaviors, or whose nonconforming gender identity or performance, has led to their being rejected or not accepted by their parents (Eliason, 2014).

OVERVIEW OF ABFT-SGM

ABFT-SGM is a systematic, empirically informed, LGBTQ+-affirmative, experiential, emotion-focused, and family-based treatment. The model is rooted in attachment theory (Bowlby, 1988), research on young adult–parent relationships (Arnett, 2014; Fingerman et al., 2012), research on parental rejection and acceptance of LGBTQ+ young adults (Kibrik et al., 2019; Ryan et al., 2009, 2010), emotion theory (Safran & Greenberg, 1991), and multidimensional family therapy (Liddle, 2009). ABFT-SGM is an adaptation of attachment-based family therapy (ABFT) for depressed adolescents (G. S. Diamond et al., 2014).

The treatment comprises five treatment tasks (see Figure 1.1), typically completed in sequence over the course of between 16 and 26 weeks. The first task is to establish relationship building as the shared goal of therapy. This task begins by connecting family members to their loss, grief, regret, and longing associated with the rupture or loss of their relationships and the

FIGURE 1.1. Overall Structure of ABFT-SGM

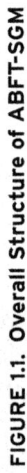

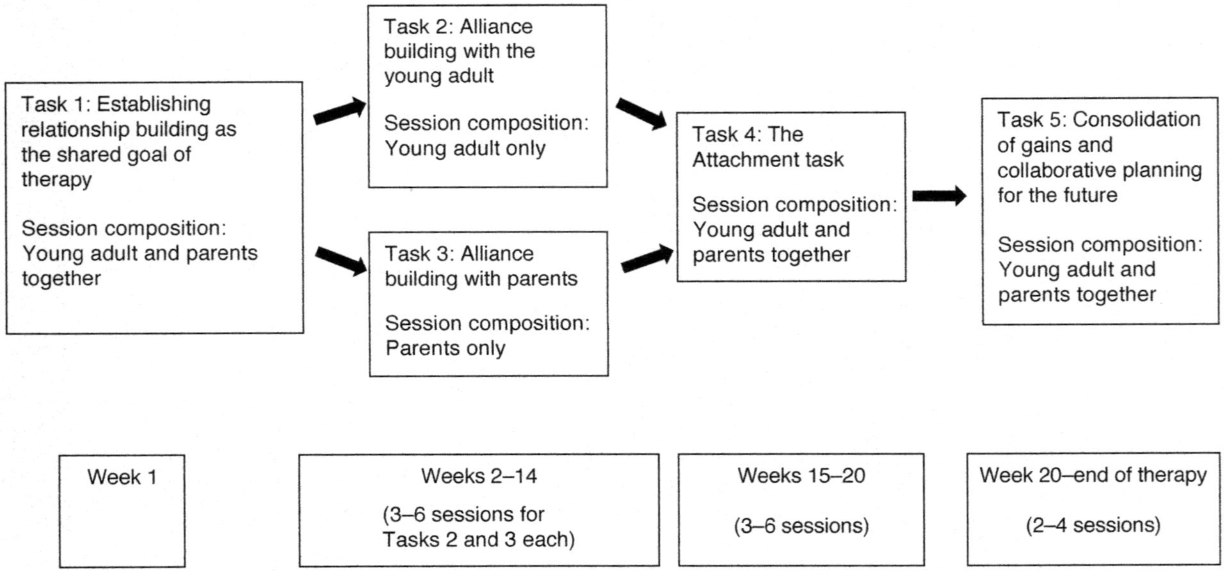

Task 1: Establishing relationship building as the shared goal of therapy

Session composition: Young adult and parents together

Task 2: Alliance building with the young adult

Session composition: Young adult only

Task 3: Alliance building with parents

Session composition: Parents only

Task 4: The Attachment task

Session composition: Young adult and parents together

Task 5: Consolidation of gains and collaborative planning for the future

Session composition: Young adult and parents together

Week 1

Weeks 2–14
(3–6 sessions for Tasks 2 and 3 each)

Weeks 15–20
(3–6 sessions)

Week 20—end of therapy
(2–4 sessions)

Note. ABFT-SGM = attachment-based family therapy for sexual and gender minority young adults and their nonaccepting parents.

fear that things may never change. Once they are connected with their loss, pain, fear, and longing, the therapist offers treatment as an opportunity for things to be different. For parents, the therapy is presented as an opportunity to work through their fear, anger, shame, and grief and to find a way, at their own pace, to become positively involved in their child's life again. For the young adult, treatment is presented as an opportunity to be heard, understood, validated, supported, and prized for who they are. For both the young adult and their parents, the opportunity to repair their bond and stay connected in a meaningful, loving, mutually respectful manner touches a deep emotional chord and existential need, and it becomes the shared goal for treatment.

Once all family members are on board, the second task of treatment is to form a strong therapeutic alliance with the young adult. To this end, the therapist meets alone with the young adult for a number of sessions. During these individual sessions, the therapist helps the young adult to connect with, and put into words, their emotions (e.g., anger, fear, sadness) associated with past and current ruptures in the relationship. These ruptures may be the result of past traumatic events (e.g., being told to not come home until they "turn straight again") or ongoing, frustrating, invalidating interactions (e.g., fights about parents' homophobic comments, parents' unwillingness to include their young adult's partner in family events). Once the young adult is fully connected with their emotions, the therapist then helps them to access and articulate their associated unmet attachment and identity needs (e.g., the need to be heard, taken seriously, respected, loved and prized for who they are). At the end of these individual sessions, the therapist prepares the young adult to share these emotions and needs directly with their parents in subsequent conjoint attachment sessions. The goal is to help the young adult share these feelings and needs with parents in a manner that will make it most likely that they will be heard. In other words, to help them share their feelings and needs in a regulated, nonattacking manner and from a place of vulnerability, while simultaneously asserting healthy boundaries.

Concurrently, the therapist meets with parents alone for several sessions. The goal of these sessions, the third task of the treatment, is to build a strong therapeutic alliance with each parent. During these sessions, the therapist helps parents access and work through their shame, grief, anger, and fear associated with their young adult's sexual orientation or gender identity. The therapist also invites parents to reflect on how their feelings and responses to their young adult's sexual orientation or gender identity have negatively affected their child and their relationship with them. As parents begin to connect to, and empathize with, their young adult's hurt, fear, anger, and loss associated with feeling rejected, parents' natural instinct to protect and care for their young adult is activated. They become motivated to better understand and support their young adult. Once parents have softened, are better able to reflect on how their nonacceptance affects their young adult and the relationship, and are motivated to do better, the therapist reintroduces relational repair as the goal of treatment. The therapist presents the therapy as an opportunity for parents to listen to, and emotionally be there for, their young adult in a manner that they have not been previously. The therapist systematically prepares the parents to respond to their young adult's feelings and needs in a more attuned manner during subsequent conjoint attachment episodes. More specifically, parents are coached to remain nondefensive, open, curious, empathic, and validating as their young adult shares their pain and adaptive needs for acceptance and connection directly with them.

The fourth task of treatment is the attachment task. During these conjoint sessions, the young adult is helped to express—directly to their parents—their hurt, fear, frustration, and anger associated with their parents' rejection/nonacceptance as well as their longing to be recognized, validated, prized, loved, and respected. The young adult is helped to communicate these feelings from a place of vulnerability and in a regulated, respectful manner. At the same time, parents are helped to respond in a nondefensive, empathic manner. As a result, the young adult feels heard, understood, and validated—often for the first time. This sense of feeling heard, understood, cared for, and safe leads the young adult to further disclose vulnerable feelings and needs. This iterative cycle of disclosure and vulnerability on the part of the young adult, and empathy, validation, concern, and support on the part of parents, leads to a reduction in tension, productive processing of grief and anger about past injuries, and a sense of trust and relief. In some cases, parents show remorse and offer an apology for having hurt their young adult. They may also take ownership of their own fears and internal conflicts associated with their young adult's identity. At the end of such episodes, family members tend to feel closer, more tender and compassionate toward one another, more mutually accepting, and more connected. Such corrective attachment episodes are considered the primary change mechanism of the therapy.

In the fifth and final task, after much of the tension in the relationship has been resolved and trust and intimacy have increased, parents and their young adult revel in the gains they have made in their relationship. They are also freed to work collaboratively to navigate the often scary next steps of living fuller, more open, and authentic lives. This may include planning together how parents will finally come out to their own parents (i.e., the grandparents), extended family members, friends, or community members.

They might also discuss when and how to invite their son's romantic partner to dinner for the first time. Conversations during this fifth task may also focus on strategies for how family members can avoid conflicts or misunderstandings in the future. For example, family members may use this task to plan how to have difficult or emotionally laden conversations when new issues come up after the treatment has ended.

In ABFT-SGM, each task builds on the previous tasks. For example, the therapist must be sure that each family member is sufficiently signed on to the goal of having difficult conversations in the therapy room before bringing them together for conjoint attachment sessions. Sometimes a task will take one or two sessions to complete; other times, it might take five or six sessions. In some cases, the therapist will want to meet with the young adult alone for an extended number of sessions because the young adult is highly anxious about directly expressing their feelings and needs to their parents. In other cases, the therapist might decide to meet with parents alone for an extended number of sessions because the parents are highly distressed and not yet in a position to hear their young adult's feelings and unmet needs. In yet other cases, the therapist may begin the attachment task only to realize that the parents or the young adult are not sufficiently on board with the treatment goal or perhaps are having a hard time regulating themselves and remaining open. In such instances, the therapist may decide to go back to meeting with family members alone to shore up the therapeutic alliance and better prepare them before resuming the conjoint attachment task. In that sense, the treatment is flexible and responsive to each family's unique needs and therapeutic process.

Although ABFT-SGM does not follow a strict protocol, the treatment does have a clear framework. The successful completion of one task sets the stage for the following task. Also, each task has its own structure with a well-articulated, detailed sequence of microsteps or subtasks. This provides the therapist with a road map and compass, directing them to where they need to go next. It also provides therapists with signposts to evaluate where they are in the treatment process. In that sense, the treatment is systematic and intentional, helping therapists to make moment-by-moment decisions in the room. At any given moment, the therapist knows what the next step is and why they have chosen to use one intervention instead of another or focus on one topic or process instead of another. For example, the therapist will know why, at a particular moment, they chose to shift from asking the young adult about how they feel when their father makes homophobic comments to asking the father how he feels hearing how hurt his child is when he makes those comments. At the same time, the flow of the session is organic and natural. The therapist intuitively feels the undercurrents of each family member's emotional world and skillfully moves the process forward in a responsive manner.

The therapist is the one with the map in hand, and they are responsible for leading the family through this landscape. They are empathic and sensitive while, at the same time, steadfast in keeping family members focused on the core, meaningful, but often difficult and painful topics at hand. They are respectful of family members' ambivalence and fears but do not acquiesce. In that sense, ABFT-SGM is best defined as client sensitive rather than client centered. The therapist's role is to guide and support family members as they walk down this path together. That said, the manner in which the therapy unfolds is based on the unique characteristics of each family. Although the structure of the treatment tasks and processes are generally the same across cases, the pace, crossroads, twists, and turns will be different for each family.

When first learning ABFT-SGM, most therapists feel awkward. This is natural and expected whenever one learns a new skill or approach. But once therapists learn the model and have treated a family or two, they typically feel a sense of excitement. They feel like they finally have a clear, coherent theory of change and a systematic practical map for how to repair or improve family relationships. In our trainings, we (GMD and RBZ) frequently hear feedback to the effect of the following:

> I do many of the things that you are talking about and have showed me. But now, I am able to put it all together. I know what I am trying to do, where I want to help the family get to, what the next step in the treatment needs to be, and how to go about it.

CORE FEATURES OF ABFT-SGM

This section describes some of the core features of ABFT-SGM. It highlights how the treatment is LGBTQ+ affirmative, relationship focused, noncoercive, and developmentally and culturally sensitive.

LGBTQ+ Affirmative

ABFT-SGM is an LGBTQ+-affirmative therapy. We, as therapists, respect and honor the young adult's lived experience and how they make meaning of that experience. We adopt the language the young adult uses to describe themselves. ABFT-SGM therapists are committed to helping young adults live as openly and authentically as they choose. Also, we do not view the relationship between parents and their young adults as symmetrical.

The treatment is founded on an explicit ethical position that parents have a fundamental responsibility to help their young adult become who they are and want to be, to feel safe in the world, and to be proud of themselves and their accomplishments. It is not the role of the young adult to fulfill their parents' dreams and expectations. Although we do take the position that young adults should treat their parents with compassion and respect, and consider their parents' values, needs, sensitivities, and limitations as they make decisions and move forward, the primary goal of the treatment is to help parents better understand; respect; and, when possible, embrace and affirm their young adult's identity.

Attachment as a Driving Motivation

A basic assumption in ABFT-SGM is that regardless of their age, deep down, young adults yearn to be seen, understood, prized, loved, respected, and supported by their parents, even if those feelings and longings have been buried under years of hurt and frustration. ABFT-SGM therapists also assume that, deep down, parents want their young adult to be happy, safe, and successful in life. That they want to support, guide, and encourage them as well as take joy in their growth, independence, and achievements.

This is true even for parents who, at the start of treatment, are highly distressed, rejecting, and avoidant. We attribute parents' nonacceptance to fear, not malice. We assume that parents who come to us for therapy love their young adult and want the best for them; that they want to do better but either do not know how or are too scared to take the steps they know they need to take.

Noncoercive

ABFT-SGM should in no way be coercive. From the outset of treatment, therapists make it clear to parents that we respect their values, religious beliefs, and customs. We do not try to force parents to become more accepting of their young adult's sexual or gender identity than they feel like they can or want to be, nor do we judge their attitudes or behaviors. Instead, we present treatment as an opportunity for parents to explore their experience of having an LGBTQ+ young adult as well as how their attitudes and behaviors have affected their young adult and their relationship with them.

ABFT-SGM is a chance for parents to reach out and hear their young adult's experience and help their young adult to feel heard, respected, and connected for the sake of both their young adult and for the relationship.

While most parents do become less rejecting and more accepting over the course of treatment, some do not. In some cases, parents become better able to hear and validate their young adult's legitimate needs but still feel unable to meet those needs (such as referring to their young adult using their chosen name and preferred pronouns). In such cases, the treatment focuses on how to create safer, more caring, and mutually respectful relationships while helping the young adult mourn and let go of some of their unfulfilled hopes.

Developmentally Sensitive

ABFT-SGM for LGBTQ+ young adults and their nonaccepting parents is an adaptation of ABFT for depressed adolescents, (G. S. Diamond et al., 2014). Such an adaptation was needed, in part, because young adults are in a different developmental stage than are adolescents, and the nature of their relationships with their parents is quite different. Whereas adolescents are typically still living with their parents, are financially dependent on them, and are subject to their parents' rules and monitoring, young adults have usually left home. In most cases, they have begun to take on the tasks of adulthood, such as forging a career path; gaining financial independence; establishing a peer support network; and, perhaps, forming meaningful romantic relationships with significant others.

Because young adults are financially, behaviorally, and psychologically more autonomous than adolescents, and further along in their identity development (including their sexual and gender identity development), the power dynamics in the relationship change. Young adults are usually more confident about who they are and what they need. This frees them to be vulnerable and express their unmet needs to be cared for, recognized, and appreciated in ways that adolescents often cannot do. At the same time, they are better able to set limits. They are less afraid of being engulfed and losing their separateness. They are able to express their feelings and needs while simultaneously seeing their parents as independent people in their own right. This leads to more mutually respectful and collaborative relationships (Koepke & Denissen, 2012). Current research findings regarding the nature of young adult–parent relationships inform the goals of ABFT-SGM.

Culture and Context

To be effective, ABFT-SGM must be delivered in a manner that is sensitive to the racial, ethnic, cultural, and religious identities and experiences of the young adult and their family. Therapy with a White evangelical family from Alabama whose gay young adult son still lives close to home and has not yet come out to his extended family will likely look different from therapy with a Black liberal family from Chicago whose genderqueer young adult is living openly in New York City and is an activist for LGBTQ+ rights. In Israel, work with an ultraorthodox Jewish family from Jerusalem will look different from work with a secular liberal family from Tel Aviv. Cultural factors influence family values and goals as well as which issues and processes are more or less salient in each case. In some cases, conversations might focus on family members' reconciling their religious beliefs with their love for their young adult and desire to have them closer. In other families, issues such as parents' standing in their community, fear of social exclusion, and shame are front and center. In yet other cases, conversations revolve around the safety and welfare of the young adult and social justice.

With racial and ethnic minority families, ABFT-SGM therapists explore the effects of bearing multiple stigmatized, deprivileged identities. For example, people of color often face both racial discrimination and heterosexism/cissexism in their everyday lives as well as racial discrimination in LGBTQ+ spaces (Balsam et al., 2011; McConnell et al., 2018). Intersectionality theory (Crenshaw, 1991), rooted in Black feminist experiences and thought, provides a helpful lens through which to examine how various forms of discrimination (e.g., racial, ethnic, religious, heterosexism, transphobia) overlap for people with multiple marginalized identities, leaving them disempowered, alienated, and vulnerable in the different arenas of their lives. For example, in Israel, an Arab Muslim lesbian is likely to feel marginalized and vulnerable for being Arab when in her apartment in Haifa and in predominately Jewish LGBTQ+ spaces, and marginalized for being LGBTQ+ when visiting the Arab village in which she was raised and her family of origin still resides.

Talking about the young adult's experience of being discriminated against and alienated in multiple systems as well as the challenges they face attempting to integrate the different and seemingly conflicting aspects of themselves (e.g., being an orthodox Jew and being gay) is important. Such conversations help parents better understand what their young adult is up against. Talking about these things can elicit parental compassion, empathy, and motivation to better support and protect their young adult. It can also help parents better see and admire their young adult's strengths, values, resilience, and sense of agency (Harvey & Stone Fish, 2015). Likewise, speaking openly with parents about their own struggle to reconcile their religious beliefs and racial and ethnic identity with being the parent of an LGBTQ+ young adult is essential to the process of facilitating acceptance and deepening the connection between parents and their young adult.

ABFT was originally developed while working with primarily urban, economically disadvantaged African American and multiracial depressed and suicidal adolescents and their families (G. Diamond et al., 2003; G. M. Diamond et al., 2012). A number of papers have since been published that illustrate how cultural factors are explicitly considered in ABFT with racial and ethnic minority lesbian, gay, and bisexual adolescents (Ibrahim et al., 2018; Levy et al., 2016). In recent years, our (GMD and RBZ's) team in Israel has worked primarily with White and Brown middle-class Israeli Jewish families. Some of these families were secular; others were religious. Some lived in large urban centers; others lived in more conservative suburban or rural communities. Most of the clinical examples in this book come from our work with these young adults and their parents. Although the guiding principles of the treatment, overall treatment goals and tasks, and therapist intervention strategies are similar across populations, the family's race, ethnicity, religious beliefs, and community milieu make each case unique.

Acceptance as a Continuum

ABFT-SGM therapists understand that different parents begin treatment at different points on the acceptance continuum. Even in the same family, two parents may be in very different spots in terms of their level of acceptance and the way that they cope with their young adult's minority identity. Parents may also have different treatment goals and levels of motivation. Therefore, what might be considered a successful treatment outcome varies greatly, depending on the given family or parent.

For example, in the case of a father who begins therapy proclaiming that he is a sworn homophobe and that nothing is going to make him believe that homosexuality is natural, a good outcome might be his being able to hear and appreciate how hurtful his homophobic comments are to his son, empathize with his son's feelings, and commit to being more careful when speaking. At the other end of the continuum might be a father who begins treatment by stating that he accepts his daughter's same-sex orientation and does not understand why she feels unheard, invalidated, or alone. In such a case, a good outcome might involve a series of heartfelt conversations during which the daughter recounts moments or interactions in which she felt hurt or invalidated, and the father responds by earnestly trying to understand, self-reflect, take responsibility, and explore what he can do so that his daughter does not feel that way in the future.

Importantly, for families that begin treatment on the more rejecting, cut-off, or conflictual end of the spectrum, what may seem like small steps toward more tolerant, open, safe, and caring relationships can be as meaningful to the young adult as the types of dramatic shifts sometimes seen in families that began treatment further along on the acceptance continuum. No matter where families begin their journey, even just a couple steps forward can mean the world.

SCOPE AND LIMITATIONS OF ABFT-SGM

A number of caveats should be kept in mind regarding the scope and limitations of ABFT-SGM.

Focused Treatment

ABFT-SGM is a focused family-based treatment specifically designed to promote parental acceptance and improve young adult–parent relationships. The treatment is not meant to be a panacea—a solution for every presenting problem. Some of the family members who come to us for therapy are facing an array of life challenges that cannot be fully addressed in the context of ABFT-SGM. For example, some parents present with high levels of marital distress: conflicts that preceded and are rooted in dynamics unrelated to their young adult's coming out. Other parents may have a history of mental health challenges, such as a history of severe depression. Some young adults may be struggling with untreated social anxiety, complex trauma, or substance abuse. Other young adults are grappling with body issues; intimacy issues; or, more generally, figuring out who they are and what they want in life.

When indicated, therapists will help family members find support and guidance beyond the context of ABFT-SGM. Sometimes this means helping them find an individual therapist, a couples therapist, or other professionals with whom to consult either before the treatment begins, while they are participating in ABFT-SGM, or after the treatment ends. Although ABFT-SGM is often conducted as a stand-alone intervention, in many cases, it is delivered as part of a more extensive, broader treatment plan.

Designed to Treat Ongoing Parental Rejection

ABFT-SGM was designed for, and tested with, families in which parents continue to reject their young adult's sexual or gender identity months or years after learning of their young adult's identity. ABFT-SGM is not necessarily the intervention that families need just after their young adult has come out for the first time. For some parents, the period immediately after their young adult comes out is emotionally charged and turbulent. They may be shocked, confused, terrified, and generally overwhelmed. What many of these parents primarily need during this period is support, validation, normalization of their feelings, psychoeducation, and reassurance that things will become more manageable with time. They need to regain their equilibrium, down-regulate, use their natural support systems, read, and educate themselves. In most cases, parents' natural coping mechanisms kick in. They quickly gain perspective, and the welfare of their child takes front and center. With the support of accepting extended family and friends, and by keeping in mind the larger picture, most families find their way back to each other without the need for therapy.

Many parents find support groups, such as PFLAG, to be beneficial during this process. Others turn to family therapists who have experience helping families navigate the coming out process. Indeed, a number of excellent books and articles provide wonderful clinical guidance for family therapists working with families during the initial coming out stage (e.g., Harvey & Stone Fish, 2015; LaSala, 2010; Savin-Williams, 2001; Stone Fish & Harvey, 2005). However, for those parents who remain stuck in their shame, fear, anger, and sense of loss—sometimes even years after their young adult's coming out— a more focused treatment, such as ABFT-SGM, may be a good option.

OVERVIEW OF THE BOOK

This book is intended for master's- and doctoral-level clinicians who have at least some training and experience in family therapy. This is not an introduction to family therapy. Delivering this treatment also requires that therapists have at least basic knowledge about sexual orientation, gender identity, sexual and gender identity development, and minority stress. For family therapists who are less familiar with this material and have less experience working with sexual and gender minority clients, reading and training in this field is recommended. It is also highly recommended that therapists who want to learn and practice ABFT-SGM use supervision to explore their own beliefs and biases about sexual and gender minority individuals.

The next chapter presents the theoretical framework and empirical support for the model. Chapters 3 through 7 present the five tasks of the treatment and the microsteps used to navigate each task. Case examples are presented to exemplify how to conduct each task. These examples come from the families we (GMD and RBZ) and our colleagues have treated in our research studies and private practice. Family members consented to have their material included in this book, and identifying details have been altered to protect the privacy of the clients. We chose cases in which family members showed at least some progress in treatment—that is, they made at least some meaningful steps toward acceptance and relational repair. This is because it is easier to learn how to apply a model when you have examples of what it looks like when the treatment unfolds as intended. In that sense, these examples provide ideal performance maps. Chapter 8 discusses special issues that arise in working with families of sexual and gender minority young adults and their nonaccepting parents, such as addressing religious beliefs and the role of siblings in the treatment. We also discuss how to work with particularly difficult cases.

We are forever indebted to the families that agreed to participate in this project over the years. Their willingness to let us in as they struggled to make sense of and come to terms with their young adult's identity and worked to build closer, more satisfying relationships was a sacred trust. At times, we felt their frustration, fear, and despair. But mostly, we witnessed their courage, love, and dedication to each other, which was nothing short of awe inspiring. Young adults garnered the courage to open up and be vulnerable. Parents, often for the first time, listened openly, empathically, and without defending themselves. They heard and connected with their child's pain and unmet needs. During such moments, young adults felt heard, prized, connected, and protected. Sometimes we all cried. At other times, we laughed together. In most cases, families finished the therapy feeling like they had found one another again.

2

EMPIRICAL BASE OF ATTACHMENT-BASED FAMILY THERAPY FOR SEXUAL AND GENDER MINORITY YOUNG ADULTS AND THEIR NONACCEPTING PARENTS

This chapter presents the research base informing the treatment goals, purported change mechanisms, and intervention strategies of attachment-based family therapy for sexual and gender minority young adults and their nonaccepting parents (ABFT-SGM). We review relevant findings from research on parental rejection and acceptance of their young adult's sexual and gender minority identity, normative young adult development, and change processes in family-based treatments. We point out how each of these bodies of knowledge have influenced and shaped the treatment model. We also summarize the findings from studies examining the efficacy of attachment-based family therapy (ABFT) in general, and ABFT-SGM in particular.

PARENTAL REJECTION AND ACCEPTANCE OF THEIR OFFSPRING'S SEXUAL AND GENDER MINORITY IDENTITY

The pervasive and pernicious effects of parental rejection on lesbian, gay, bisexual, transgender, and queer (LGBTQ+) adolescents, emerging adults, and young adults have been well documented. A large number of studies have

https://doi.org/10.1037/0000352-002
Attachment-Based Family Therapy for Sexual and Gender Minority Young Adults and Their Nonaccepting Parents, by G. M. Diamond and R. Boruchovitz-Zamir

found that parents' rejection of their child's sexual orientation or gender identity is associated with dramatically higher rates of depression, anxiety, suicidal ideation, suicide attempts, internalized stigma, identity concealment, and rejection sensitivity (Bouris et al., 2010; D'Augelli, 2002; Grossman et al., 2021; Hall, 2018; Kiekens et al., 2020; Pachankis et al., 2008; Parra et al., 2018; Ryan et al., 2009; Tate & Patterson, 2019). These findings hold true not only in samples of predominately White people but also in samples of people of color (Mitrani et al., 2017; Salerno et al., 2022). For example, Ryan et al. (2009) conducted a seminal study on a sample of 224 Latinx and White lesbian, gay, and bisexual (LGB) emerging adults based in the United States and found that greater levels of parental sexual orientation–specific rejection during adolescence were associated with a wide range of negative mental and physical health outcomes during young adulthood, including higher rates of depression, suicide attempts, use of illicit drugs, and unprotected sex. Results from a recent cross-sectional study of 256 Israeli LGB young adults revealed that levels of parental rejection of their sexual orientation predicted the severity of their psychological symptoms, even after accounting for levels of parental global rejection (i.e., parental rejection associated with aspects of the young adult's life not related to their sexual orientation; Kibrik et al., 2019).

In one of the few longitudinal studies published to date, Pachankis et al. (2018) examined the prospective relationships among parents' rejection of their young adult's sexual orientation, the young adult's report of unfinished business (e.g., feeling frustrated about not having their needs met by their parent; feeling troubled by unresolved negative feelings in relation to their parent, such as anger, grief, hurt), and depressive symptoms. They followed a group of 113 U.S. college students for 7 years, beginning from around the age of 20. Findings showed that parental rejection of their young adult's sexual orientation predicted greater levels of young adults' unfinished business in the subsequent year, and that unfinished business with fathers, in turn, predicted young adults' depressive symptoms in the next year.

In contrast to the deleterious effects of parental rejection, parental acceptance of their child's sexual orientation and gender identity has been linked to higher levels of self-esteem, better adjustment, and lower levels of psychological distress among LGBTQ+ adolescents, emerging adults, and young adults (D'Augelli, 2002; Eisenberg & Resnick, 2006; Elizur & Ziv, 2001; Evans et al., 2004; Floyd et al., 1999; Hershberger & D'Augelli, 1995; Needham & Austin, 2010; Ryan et al., 2010; Savin-Williams, 1989; Sheets & Mohr, 2009; Shilo et al., 2015; Simons et al., 2013). For example, Ryan et al. (2010) found that greater parental acceptance of their child's sexual orientation and gender identity during adolescence was associated with a wide range of positive mental and physical health outcomes during emerging adulthood, including greater self-esteem, social support and general health, as well as lower levels of depressive symptoms and suicidal ideation. Along the same lines, Kibrik et al. (2019) found that maternal sexual orientation–specific acceptance predicted lower levels of psychological distress among a sample of Israeli LGB young adults, even after accounting for global maternal acceptance. A recent study of LGB young adults in China also found that parental sexual orientation–specific support was positively correlated with young adults' psychological adjustment (Shao et al., 2018).

Parental acceptance and support may be the *most* important source of acceptance and support for LGBTQ+ offspring. Indeed, a second study on the Ryan et al. (2010) sample found that emerging adults' retrospective reports of their parents' sexual orientation- or gender-specific acceptance during adolescence predicted their current levels of well-being and adjustment above and beyond the effects of friend and community support (Snapp et al., 2015). Likewise, in a study of Israeli LGB adolescents and emerging adults, Shilo and Savaya (2011) found that family support had a stronger effect on participants' self-acceptance than did support by friends.

It is worth noting that parental acceptance and rejection are related but not identical constructs. They are not opposite ends of the same continuum (Kibrik et al., 2019). For example, parents can become less rejecting (e.g., decrease their homophobic remarks and coercive attempts to influence their young adult's behaviors) without necessarily becoming more accepting (e.g., show more interest in their young adult's personal life, be more open with friends and family about their child's identity). Indeed, studies have shown that young adult–parent relationships characterized by low levels of both sexual orientation–specific parental acceptance and rejection are actually common (Clark et al., 2021; LaSala, 2010; Livingston & Fourie, 2016).

Informed by these research findings, ABFT-SGM therapists target both parental rejecting and accepting behaviors. Optimal treatment outcomes are characterized by not only a reduction in rejecting parental behaviors, such as explicit criticism, invalidation, coercion, and microaggressions, but also an increase in accepting and affirming parental behaviors. Such accepting and affirming parental behaviors include increasing positive involvement in their young adult's life; coming out to extended family, colleagues, and friends; working to become more comfortable around LGBTQ+ people; and advocating for social justice.

ATTACHMENT, AUTONOMY, AND RELATEDNESS IN YOUNG ADULTHOOD

ABFT-SGM is unique because it addresses parental sexual orientation and gender identity–specific rejection and acceptance in young adulthood. To fully understand the significance and implications of parental acceptance and rejection for LGBTQ+ young adults, these processes need to be examined in the context of developmental research on normative young adult–parent relationships in the general population. Healthy adaptive relationships between young adults and their parents are characterized by the coexistence of attachment, relatedness, and autonomy (Koepke & Denissen, 2012). Research shows that although physical proximity between children and their parents may decrease during young adulthood, parents still serve as primary attachment figures (Doherty & Feeney, 2004; Trinke & Bartholomew, 1997). Securely attached young adults feel like their parents will be there for them if they need them and will go to their parents for comfort and support in times of distress and need (Doherty & Feeney, 2004). Indeed, a survey by Arnett and Schwab (2012) found that the majority of U.S. young adults are in contact with their parents via text, email, or phone nearly every day. Moreover, parents provide their young adults with a wide range of types of support, including financial, instrumental, and emotional. Such support has been linked to young adults' higher life satisfaction and better adjustment (Fingerman et al., 2012).

Healthy young adult–parent relationships are also characterized by psychological autonomy. In contrast to adolescence, the power distribution in relationships between young adults and their parents is more balanced. There is mutual respect and recognition, and parents support the psychological autonomy of their young adult. They view their young adult as distinct from themselves. They see them as independent, competent people in their own right. They are curious and respectful of their young adult's opinions and values. This allows the young adult to explore who they are and who they are becoming without fear of being judged, rejected, intruded upon, controlled, or abandoned (Luyckx et al., 2007). Such exploration allows young adults to increasingly see themselves as a separate person with their own identity. At the same time, young adults have an increasingly realistic appraisal of parents as individual persons having both strengths and weaknesses. Optimal identity development in young adulthood does not occur in isolation from parents but, rather, within the context of a "we" relationship with their parents (Koepke & Denissen, 2012).

Increased behavioral autonomy is another hallmark of healthy young adult–parent relationships. In contrast to adolescents, most emerging and young adults live outside of the home. Parents have less control over the choices their young adult makes and less ability to monitor those choices. This allows young adults added degrees of freedom to operate in the world as they continue discovering who they are and what they want in life. At the same time, young adulthood means transitioning into adult roles with greater responsibilities. This includes making career choices with long-lasting implications; becoming more independent financially; and, perhaps, choosing a life partner and starting a family. Armed with greater clarity about themselves, together with an increased sense of competence, independence, and autonomy, young adults reapproach their parents from a more confident, individuated position. This combination of secure attachment, psychological autonomy, and behavioral autonomy allows for more open, honest, egalitarian, mutual, and satisfying relationships with parents (Aquilino, 2006; Koepke & Denissen, 2012). On the whole, parents and young adults alike report that their relationships have improved since adolescence. They report that their relationships are more harmonious, honest, stronger, and enjoyable than in the past. They describe having more adult-type conversations, which lead to more intimate and meaningful connections (Arnett, 2014).

ABFT-SGM therapists keep in mind this delicate balance of attachment, autonomy, and relatedness in their work with LGBTQ+ young adults and their parents. They strive to promote continued connection while supporting good healthy boundaries. They use their knowledge of normative developmental processes to help family members form age-appropriate relationships and to set adaptive goals for the treatment. They are also aware that LGBTQ+ young adults who have grown up in nonaccepting environments may be particularly sensitive to parental invalidation and psychological control. Consequently, they work to help parents understand how invalidating their young adult's experience, denying the legitimacy of their sexual or gender identity, attempting to control their young adult's thoughts or behavior, or being unable to revel in and admire their young adult for who they are undermines their young adult's sense of self. Even as adults, we want to feel like our parents appreciate, admire, and are proud of us.

Not only does parental invalidation and controlling behavior undermine the self of the young adult, but it often leads to conflict or distance in the attachment relationship. This, in turn, makes it less likely that the young adult will receive the types of parental support, comfort, and guidance that are so important during this developmental stage. Parental support, validation, and pride may be even more important for LGBTQ+ young adults than for heteronormative, cisgender young adults because of the minority stress most LGBTQ+ people face in their personal lives and in society at large

(Meyer, 2003). For those reasons, ABFT-SGM therapists highlight themes related to attachment, autonomy, and relatedness throughout the treatment and work to promote mutual recognition, acceptance, and respect in the context of ongoing connection.

ENACTMENT AS A MECHANISM OF CHANGE

The attachment task, which comprises corrective attachment episodes, is considered the primary change mechanism in ABFT-SGM. A *corrective attachment episode* is a specific type of enactment or in-session interaction between family members. Enactments are a core element of most couples and family therapies (Gardner & Butler, 2009). When used as a therapeutic intervention, enactments are designed to help family members engage with one another in a new, more open, direct, productive, and sustained manner (Minuchin, 1974). Successful enactments transform interactional patterns, facilitate the disclosure of adaptive emotions and unmet needs, allow for the working through of past hurts and current impasses, shift perceptions of self and others, and increase trust and security in relationships (Davis & Butler, 2004; Nichols & Colapinto, 2017).

Conducting successful enactments, however, is a complicated and challenging task for therapists. Fueled by intense emotions and reactivity, couple and family interactions have the potential to escalate quickly. Family members may begin attacking one another and withdrawing. Family members may also overly focus on the concrete details of a given event (e.g., "You didn't even say anything to Dad when he made that comment about 'dykes'!") rather than connect with and express underlying feelings and core needs (e.g., "I feel alone in those moments. I need you to stand up for me"). Therefore, it is critical for therapists to have an empirically based clinical map to guide them as they work to shape enactments so that they are therapeutic and transformative.

The clinical map for conducting corrective attachment episodes in ABFT-SGM is based on findings from a number of studies. These studies used task-analytic and other change-event methodologies to identify in-session sequences of couples and family members' behaviors and affective–cognitive states associated with relational repair. For example, findings from research on emotion-focused therapy (EFT) for couples for unresolved emotional injuries showed that when one member of the couple expressed vulnerability and the other member immediately responded with expressions of support, forgiveness was facilitated and trust increased (McKinnon & Greenberg, 2017). When one of the partners had been betrayed by the other, forgiveness occurred when the offending partner assumed responsibility for the emotional injury and then expressed either shame or empathic distress, or offered a heartfelt apology, followed by the injured partner evidencing a shift in their view of the injurer (Meneses & Greenberg, 2011).

In another study on EFT for couples with an attachment injury, findings showed that such injuries were resolved in cases in which the following process occurred: The injured partner accessed and integrated disowned attachment-related emotions linked to the incident and communicated hurt and longing. The offending partner took responsibility or expressed regret and offered an apology. The injured partner accepted the apology, expressing vulnerable emotions and attachment needs, and the offending partner responded to their partner's feelings and needs in an empathic and responsive manner. Key therapist interventions found to facilitate this process included reflecting primary emotions, evocative responding, heightening, and inviting partners to respond to the other's attachment needs and concerns about the injury at an emotional level (Zuccarini et al., 2013).

In a seminal study on enactments in family therapy, Friedlander et al. (1994) examined how family members participating in structural family therapy remained productively engaged with one another (i.e., willingly shared their thoughts and feelings, cooperated, were responsive and attentive to one another) for a sustained amount of time. They found that sustained engagement occurred when family members acknowledged their own contribution to the impasse, communicated their thoughts and feelings about the impasse to the other, acknowledged the thoughts and feelings of the other, evidenced shifts in their attributions regarding the other's behaviors, and recognized the benefits of resolving the impasse.

In a study on resolving impasses in multidimensional family therapy for adolescent substance abusers (G. Diamond & Liddle, 1996), successful resolution occurred when the following happened: The blaming parent verbalized regret or sadness, and the adolescent was surprised but encouraged. The parent then showed curiosity about their adolescent's experience. The adolescent expressed feelings of vulnerability and a need for closeness with their parent, and the parent expressed empathy. The adolescent expressed legitimate assertive anger about past attachment failures, and the parent took responsibility for their part. Importantly, the authors found that therapists held a central role in orchestrating the resolution sequence. Therapists actively blocked, diverted, or helped family members work through their negative affect, mutual blame, and helplessness while evoking, amplifying, and punctuating decreases in hostility or defensiveness and increases in parental curiosity, caring, and sadness.

Two studies have examined the process of repairing attachment in ABFT. The first examined the attachment task in ABFT for depressed adolescents. Results showed that in successful attachment sessions, parents showed more respect for their adolescent's experience, evidenced warmth and empathy, took responsibility for their part in the relational rupture, and apologized. Adolescents, for their part, more directly expressed their feelings and needs. In contrast, in unsuccessful attachment tasks, parents were belittling and blaming, and they sulked (G. S. Diamond & Stern, 2003).

The second study examined corrective attachment episodes in ABFT for young adults presenting with unresolved anger toward their parent (Tsvieli et al., 2022). Findings revealed two multistep sequences reflective of good outcome cases. At the beginning of the first sequence, the therapist focused on the young adult's primary adaptive emotions, and the young adult productively processed their vulnerable emotions. Then, the therapist empathized with and validated the parent as they listened to their child, followed by the parent's expression of warmth toward their young adult. In the second sequence, the therapist first focused on the young adult's unmet attachment needs, and the young adult productively processed their vulnerable emotions. Then, the parent expressed a willingness to fulfill their young adult's attachment needs followed by an expression of warmth toward their young adult. These findings illustrate the circular, iterative, in-session sequences of therapist interventions, young adults' disclosure of vulnerable emotions and unmet needs, and parents' empathic and validating responses that, together, lead to increased trust and safety in the young adult–parent relationship, resolution of anger, and decreases in psychological symptoms (G. S. Diamond et al., 2014; Kobak & Bosmans, 2019).

On the whole, these findings provide a robust clinical map for ABFT-SGM therapists as they work toward facilitating relational repair. It appears that one essential component of the process is helping parents to reach out to their young adult from a place of warmth, empathy, and curiosity and invite them to share their feelings and needs. Another component is facilitating the young adult's productive emotional processing and, in particular, their sharing of adaptive vulnerable emotions. Finally, therapists need to help parents listen to and validate their young adult's experience, take responsibility for things they have done that have hurt their child, and connect with their own empathic distress when witnessing their young adult's pain.

THE ROLE OF YOUNG ADULTS' PRODUCTIVE EMOTIONAL PROCESSING IN ABFT-SGM

In light of the purported role that young adults' vulnerability plays in the change process, two studies directly examined the link between productive emotional processing and treatment outcome. The first study explored the association between emotional processing and treatment outcome in a sample of 39 suicidal adolescents who had received 16 weeks of ABFT (Lifshitz et al., 2021). It examined theoretically driven sequential pathways through which adolescents were expected to traverse as they moved from secondary global distress and rejecting anger to primary adaptive hurt, grief, and assertive anger. As hypothesized, adolescents moved from states of global distress to maladaptive shame, from maladaptive rejecting anger to adaptive assertive anger, and from adaptive assertive anger to adaptive grief/hurt, although these sequences were not unique to cases with good treatment outcomes. Poorer treatment outcome was, however, associated with higher rates of adolescents' maladaptive global distress.

The second study explored the link between the amount of young adults' productive emotional processing and treatment outcome in ABFT and EFT for young adults presenting with unresolved anger toward their parent (G. M. Diamond et al., 2016). Emotional processing was measured during attachment sessions (in the ABFT condition) or during empty-chair interventions (in the EFT condition). Results showed that the amount of young adults' productive emotional processing predicted pre- to posttherapy changes in psychological symptoms in both treatments, although it did not predict decreases in unresolved anger, state anger, or attachment anxiety and avoidance in either condition.

PROMOTING YOUNG ADULTS' PRODUCTIVE EMOTIONAL PROCESSING IN ABFT-SGM

Helping young adults access their vulnerable emotions is not a trivial matter. Even in the context of therapy approaches like ABFT-SGM and EFT that focus on eliciting vulnerability, such moments are hard to come by and are often fleeting (G. M. Diamond et al., 2016; Kramer et al., 2015). To better understand which therapist interventions promote such productive emotional processing, two studies were conducted. The first study was on a sample of 30 depressed and suicidal adolescents receiving ABFT (Tsvieli et al., 2020). Sequential analyses revealed that relational reframes (i.e., shifting adolescents' focus onto the loss in their relationship with their parents) and focusing on primary adaptive emotions were associated with the subsequent initiation of adolescents' productive emotional processing of primary adaptive emotions. In contrast, interventions not intended to promote productive emotional processing, such as interpretations, reassurance, and focus on the adolescents' rejecting anger toward their parents, led to the discontinuation of adolescents' emotional processing that had already begun. Therapists' general encouragement of affect and focus on adolescents' unmet attachment/identity needs were associated with both the initiation of adolescents' productive emotional processing and the discontinuation of such processing once it had already begun.

In a second study, conducted on a sample of 15 young adults receiving ABFT for unresolved anger toward a parent, results indicated that young adults' productive emotional processing occurred at a rate significantly greater than chance following therapists' focus on vulnerable emotions and attachment needs and following empty-chair interventions. In contrast, therapists' focus on the young adult's rejecting anger preceded the discontinuation of such processing at rates significantly greater than chance (Tsvieli & Diamond, 2018).

ABFT-SGM therapists keep in mind that family members often present with secondary emotional reactions to underlying primary vulnerable emotions and that activating these secondary maladaptive emotion schema can provide access to primary adaptive vulnerable emotions (Greenberg, 2012; Pascual-Leone & Greenberg, 2007; Rochman et al., 2008). Also, a number of specific therapist interventions have been shown to be effective in helping family members access their vulnerable emotions, such as adaptive sadness and grief. These interventions include using relational reframes (i.e., shifting the client's attention to the loss in the relationship); focusing on the family member's core unmet needs; and directly asking about primary adaptive emotions, such as hurt and grief (Pascual-Leone & Kramer, 2019; Tsvieli & Diamond, 2018).

THE THERAPEUTIC ALLIANCE

ABFT-SGM emphasizes the importance of establishing a strong therapeutic alliance with all family members. This is because the *therapeutic alliance*, most commonly defined as the strength of the bond between the client and the therapist and the degree to which the client and therapist agree on the goals and tasks of treatment (Bordin, 1994), has long been recognized as an essential aspect of effective psychotherapy across a wide range of treatment approaches, including family therapy (Flückiger et al., 2018). Indeed, a number of comprehensive reviews as well as a recent meta-analysis of close to 40 independent family therapy studies have shown that the stronger the therapeutic alliance, the better the treatment outcome (Friedlander et al., 2018; Heatherington et al., 2015; Rohrbaugh, 2014).

Forming and maintaining therapeutic alliances in family therapy is complicated. Family therapy includes multiple family members who may hold conflicting or competing definitions of the problem at hand and thoughts about what needs to happen to solve the problem. They also may have varying levels of motivation, psychological mindedness, and emotion regulation capacities. The job of the therapist is to help all family members feel heard and understood and to help them reach an agreed on, shared goal of therapy. The ideal goal is something that is important to all of them and that they are willing to work toward in tandem (Friedlander et al., 2006); otherwise, family members may be working toward different ends and pulling in opposite directions.

The alliance with each family member also needs to be sufficiently strong. In family therapy, there is a danger of developing unbalanced alliances, whereby one family member feels like the therapist understands and likes them and identifies with their feelings and needs, whereas another family member feels misunderstood, neglected, and judged by the therapist. It is critical that the therapist monitor the strength of their alliance with each family member throughout the course of treatment. Research has shown that *split alliances* in which one family member reports a strong alliance with the therapist and another family member reports a weak alliance with the therapist are linked to poorer treatment outcome and premature termination (Friedlander et al., 2021).

In ABFT-SGM, the alliance is important for a number of reasons. First, it serves to soothe and engage family members. For that reason, ABFT-SGM therapists begin treatment by systematically developing a bond with each family member, starting from the first moments of the first session. They do this by empathically listening to and validating the young adult's sense of fear, anger, and grief deriving from their parents' rejecting behaviors and, at the same time, empathizing with parents' sense of fear, shame, anger, and helplessness. Such alliance building continues when, near the end of the first session, the therapist highlights the rupture in the young adult–parent relationship, amplifies the loss and pain both sides have experienced as a result of the relational rupture, and offers relationship building as a shared goal of treatment.

The second function of the alliance in ABFT-SGM is to enlist and motivate the young adult and their parents to productively partake in the tasks of the treatment, particularly the attachment task. Toward that end, the therapist concurrently meets separately with the young adult alone and with parents alone. During sessions alone with the young adult (i.e., the second task of the treatment), the therapist helps them to connect with their vulnerable emotions and unmet needs (e.g., longing for care, recognition and connection with parents), and then offers subsequent conjoint attachment sessions as an opportunity for them to communicate their feelings and unmet needs directly to their parents. During sessions alone with parents (i.e., the third task of the treatment), the therapist works to help parents reflect on their young adult's hurt and legitimate adaptive anger and enlists them in the goal of being there for their young adult in a manner that they have not been before. The therapist offers subsequent attachment episodes as an opportunity for parents to reach out to their young adult to hear—perhaps for the first time—their pain and unmet needs. In that sense, the alliance in ABFT-SGM is best conceived of as a platform from which family members engage in the work of the treatment rather than as simply a curative factor in and of itself.

One study of 19 families with a suicidal and depressed adolescent receiving ABFT (Feder & Diamond, 2016) found that the strength of the parent–therapist alliance during the alliance building with parents task predicted the degree to which parents exhibited attachment-promoting behaviors in subsequent conjoint attachment sessions. More specifically, the stronger the parent–therapist alliance, the more parents encouraged their adolescent to share their emotions and unmet needs and the more parents responded in an empathic, nondefensive, noncritical manner during subsequent conjoint attachment sessions.

In a second study, Shpigel and Diamond (2014) used a consensual qualitative research approach to examine therapeutic themes and processes uniquely associated with good versus poor therapeutic alliances with nonaccepting parents in ABFT-SGM. Results showed that in good alliances, parents adopted relationship building as a goal, considered essentialist causal attributions of same-sex orientation (e.g., sexual orientation as being biologically based and immutable), acknowledged positive aspects of their child, and perceived the therapist as empathic and accepting. In contrast, parents with poor alliances rejected relationship building as a goal, rebuffed essentialist causal attributions, dismissed the possibility of their coming out as parents of an LGBTQ+ child, nullified positive aspects of their child, sought to change their child's sexual orientation, blamed therapists for validating their child's same-sex orientation, and pressured therapists for information about their young adult.

It is worth noting that alliance building is not a one-time task and that the strength of the alliance with each family member can fluctuate over time. ABFT-SGM therapists monitor the state of the alliance with each family member over the course of therapy. When the therapist suspects that a rupture has occurred in one or more of the alliances, they will take any number of steps to repair the alliance, including asking the family member how they feel regarding the therapeutic relationship or explicitly addressing the rupture. In some instances, the therapist may choose to go back to meeting with parents or the young adult alone to explore their ambivalence, reconnect them to their pain and longing, and reestablish repairing the attachment relationship as the shared goal of treatment.

EMPIRICAL SUPPORT FOR THE EFFICACY OF ABFT FOR DEPRESSED AND SUICIDAL ADOLESCENTS AND FOR YOUNG ADULTS WITH UNRESOLVED ANGER TOWARD A PARENT

ABFT for Depressed and Suicidal Adolescents

The development and testing of ABFT began with Guy S. Diamond's seminal work at the Philadelphia Child Guidance Clinic in the late 1990s. After developing the model, he and his team conducted a series of randomized clinical trials. The first involved randomly assigning 32 adolescents diagnosed with major depressive disorder (MDD), many of whom were African American and came from low-income families, to 12 weeks of ABFT or 6 weeks of a wait-list control condition. Of the 16 treatment cases, 13 (81%) no longer met criteria for MDD at posttreatment, whereas only seven (47%) of the 15 patients on the wait-list no longer met criteria for MDD post–wait-list, a significant between-group difference. At treatment's end, 62% of the adolescents treated with ABFT had a score of 9 or less on the Beck Depression Inventory (Beck et al., 1961) compared with 19% of the adolescents in the wait-list condition. At 6-month follow-up, 87% of the treated sample no longer met criteria for MDD and showed significant reductions in depression, anxiety, and family conflict as well as improvements in family cohesion (G. S. Diamond et al., 2002).

The second clinical trial (G. S. Diamond et al., 2010) involved randomizing 66 depressed and suicidal adolescents to 16 weeks of either ABFT or enhanced usual care (EUC). EUC involved assisting families in obtaining a therapist in the community, developing a safety plan, conducting weekly tracking of depression and suicidal ideation, and providing access to a 24-hour crisis line. Compared with EUC, youth treated with ABFT exhibited significantly greater and faster reductions in suicidal ideation during treatment. These differences persisted at follow-up, with a large effect size of .97. ABFT was even effective with the most severe youth—those presenting with comorbid anxiety, a history of multiple suicide attempts, or a history of sexual abuse (G. Diamond et al., 2012). Results also indicated that ABFT was associated with greater rates of clinical recovery and treatment retention. At post-treatment, 87% of patients receiving ABFT reported suicidal ideation scores not only below the clinical cutoff, but also in a range consistent with or below that of a nonclinical sample of similar demographics (Reynolds & Mazza, 1999). For EUC, only 51% achieved this level of recovery. Benefits were maintained at follow-up with a strong effect size ($OR = 4.41$).

The third randomized clinical trial (G. S. Diamond et al., 2019) compared ABFT for suicidal and depressed adolescents with family-enhanced non-directive supportive therapy (FE-NST; Brent & Kolko, 1991). Adolescents in the ABFT condition showed significant reductions in suicidal ideation, with an effect size of $d = 2.24$. Adolescents in the FE-NST condition experienced a similar significant reduction, with an effect size of $d = 1.93$. Response rates (i.e., 50% or more reduction in suicide ideation symptoms from baseline) at posttreatment were 69.1% for ABFT versus 62.3% for FE-NST. Similar results were found for depressive symptoms.

ABFT for LGBTQ+ Depressed and Suicidal Adolescents

The large number of sexual minority adolescents presenting in earlier clinical trials led the research team at the Center for Family Intervention Studies to adapt ABFT to the unique needs of LGB adolescents and their parents and then research the adapted model. In Phase I of the study (G. M. Diamond et al., 2012), a group of experts met to modify the treatment. Adaptations included (a) spending more individual time working with caregivers to process their disappointment, pain, anger, and fear related to their adolescent's minority sexual identity; (b) addressing the meaning, implications, and process of acceptance for both caregivers and adolescents; and (c) increasing caregivers' awareness of their subtle yet potent invalidating responses to their adolescents' sexual identity (i.e., microaggressions). After adapting the treatment, G. M. Diamond et al. (2012) conducted an open pilot trial in which 10 LGB depressed and suicidal adolescents and their parents received 12 weeks of therapy. Results showed that those adolescents who completed treatment reported significant decreases in suicidal ideation, depressive symptoms, and maternal attachment–related anxiety and avoidance, with medium to large effect sizes.

Recently, Russon et al. (2021) tested the feasibility, acceptability, and preliminary effectiveness of ABFT when delivered in LGBTQ+ community settings. Ten participants were enrolled in 16 weeks of ABFT across three LGBTQ+ organizations. Eight of the 10 adolescents identified as transgender or gender diverse. ABFT was found to be both feasible and acceptable. All participants completed treatment. Adolescents and their caregivers reported high therapeutic alliance scores throughout treatment. There was a significant decrease in suicidal ideation but not depression.

ABFT for Young Adults With Unresolved Anger Toward a Parent

ABFT has also been adapted for, and implemented with, emerging and young adults presenting with unresolved anger toward their parents, independent of their sexual orientation or gender. In a clinical trial comparing ABFT with individual EFT (Greenberg, 2011), 32 participants received 10 weeks of therapy. Results showed that although both treatments led to significant and equivalent decreases in anger resolution, state anger, attachment anxiety, and psychological symptoms, only ABFT was associated with a decrease in attachment avoidance (G. M. Diamond et al., 2016).

THE ABFT-SGM MODEL

The clinical model presented in this book is informed primarily from the work my colleagues and I (GMD) have done over the past 10 years adapting ABFT for sexual and gender minority young adults and their nonaccepting parents (G. M. Diamond et al., 2019). Like ABFT for young adults with unresolved anger, ABFT-SGM does not primarily focus on reducing psychological symptoms (e.g., suicidal ideation, depressive symptoms); rather, this model focuses on reducing parental rejection, increasing parental acceptance, and improving the quality of the young adult–parent attachment relationship. These are the primary outcome targets of the treatment.

In a just completed open trial, we (G. M. Diamond et al., 2022) provided 30 Israeli LGBTQ+ young adults and their nonaccepting parents with up to 26 weeks of ABFT-SGM. Multilevel multivariate growth analyses revealed that both young adults and their parents independently reported increases in parents' acceptance of the young adult's same-sex orientation or noncisgender identity. In addition, young adults reported decreases in parents' levels of rejection. Also, mothers, but not fathers, reported decreases in their own levels of rejection. Finally, young adults reported a decrease in attachment avoidance in their relationships with both mothers and fathers but not a decrease in attachment anxiety. Importantly, these treatment gains were maintained at 3 months follow-up.

In a separate process study on this same sample, Boruchovitz-Zamir and Diamond (2019) examined changes in parents' in-session behaviors during conjoint sessions over the course of the treatment and whether such changes were correlated with young adults' experience of parental acceptance and rejection. Parents' behaviors were measured via observer ratings. Findings revealed that reductions in parents' negative behaviors (e.g., criticism, invalidation) predicted decreases in young adults' self-reports of perceived parental rejection of their identity (Boruchovitz-Zamir & Diamond, 2019).

To summarize, support for the efficacy of ABFT for young adults in general, and for ABFT-SGM for LGBTQ+ young adults in particular, is accruing. More studies with larger samples and active control conditions are needed. That said, the evidence gathered so far is promising. Likewise, ABFT-SGM researchers at Ben-Gurion University are gaining more and more insight into the mechanisms associated with good outcome in ABFT-SGM as well as the therapist interventions that promote such processes. Change processes, such as the development of a strong therapeutic alliance, young adults' productive emotional processing, parental reflective functioning, and an increase in parental validating and empathic responses, warrant further attention by researchers.

3 ESTABLISHING RELATIONSHIP BUILDING AS THE SHARED GOAL OF THERAPY

The first task of attachment-based family therapy for sexual and gender minority young adults and their nonaccepting parents (ABFT-SGM) is to establish relationship building as the focus and shared goal of treatment. This task is conducted during the initial session of therapy, which includes both the young adult and their parents. The therapist begins by orienting the family to the treatment and then briefly getting to know each family member (see Figure 3.1). Once family members feel comfortable, and an initial bond has been formed, the conversation turns to what brought them to treatment. Young adults typically share feelings of frustration, anger, hurt, and sadness in the face of their parents' nonacceptance. They talk about wanting their parents to be interested in their lives; to accept, love, admire, and respect them for who they are; and to support their efforts to live openly and proudly. They also talk about wanting to feel like they are part of the family. Parents, on the other hand, typically share feeling confused, helpless, ashamed, and afraid in regard to their young adult's sexual orientation or gender identity. They talk about their struggle to reconcile their hetero- and gender-normative expectations and cultural and religious beliefs with the reality of having a sexual or gender minority young adult child.

https://doi.org/10.1037/0000352-003
Attachment-Based Family Therapy for Sexual and Gender Minority Young Adults and Their Nonaccepting Parents, by G. M. Diamond and R. Boruchovitz-Zamir

FIGURE 3.1. Structure of Establishing Relationship Building as the Shared Goal of Therapy Task

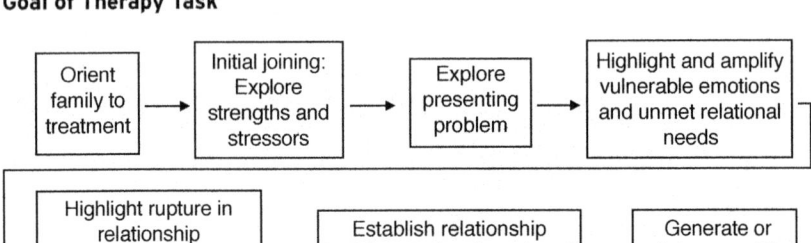

After hearing from all family members, the therapist focuses on and amplifies the young adult's experience of fear, hurt, and loss. They also mark the shared grief both the young adult and their parents are experiencing because of the rupture in their relationship. Once family members' distress is sufficiently manifested and the cost of parents' nonacceptance is clear, the therapist offers ABFT-SGM as a way out of their misery. To the young adult, the therapist presents treatment as a chance to be heard, understood, validated, or at least respected and safe. To parents, treatment is presented as an opportunity to work through their own shame, fear, anger, confusion, and grief so that they can be closer with, and more responsive to, their young adult—even if they are not yet able to fully accept their young adult's sexual or gender minority identity. To the family as a whole, treatment is presented as an opportunity to form warmer, more loving, open, honest, trusting, mutually respectful relationships and to remain connected.

BEGINNING THERAPY

The therapy begins by meeting with the young adult and their parents together for a first conjoint session. The immediate task at hand is to help each family member feel comfortable. Therefore, therapists start by introducing themselves and then checking in to see how each family member is doing as they arrive to the office for the first time. In these initial moments, family members often need to settle down from the hustle and bustle of life. They may be understandably anxious about coming to a new setting, meeting an unfamiliar therapist, and not knowing what to expect from the treatment.

Once the family members have settled in, the therapist makes sure to acknowledge their willingness to participate in the treatment. We do this because coming to therapy, and family therapy in particular, can be scary. It takes courage. The young adults who come to us do so facing the risk that if they open up and allow themselves to be vulnerable, they may end up getting hurt again and feeling even more frustrated, disconnected, and hopeless. Parents, for their part, may fear being blamed or attacked. They may also fear talking about things that are painful or make them feel guilty, inadequate, or ashamed. Parents may also worry that we, the therapists, will identify more with their young adult than with them. They may suspect that we do not understand, care about, or empathize with how difficult it has been for them coming to terms with having a sexual or gender minority young adult, or that we will not appreciate or respect their values or religious beliefs. Consequently, they may be afraid that we will judge them or push them to do things that they do not want, or feel able, to do. For all of these reasons, it is crucial that we are cognizant of and acknowledge family members' vulnerability and fears in these early moments of therapy, recognize the effort and courage needed for them to come to our offices, and create an environment of safety and nonjudgmental acceptance.

After this initial settling in, the therapist gives a brief overview of the structure of the treatment, saying something like this:

> Okay. Now that you all are here, just a few words about today's session and how the rest of the treatment will go. Today, I want to get to know each of you a little bit, above and beyond the reasons why you have come to therapy. Then, we will talk about why you came in and what you would like to get out of the treatment. Next week, I will begin meeting with you [i.e., the young adult] alone for a few sessions, and the two of you [i.e., the parents] alone for a few sessions. We will have these separate sessions in parallel. Finally, when you are all ready, we will get back together again for a number of sessions so that you all can talk about some of the things that have been bothering you and what you would like to be different in the relationship, but in a manner that feels safe and productive.

This description of the therapy structure and process is intentionally brief. It is sufficiently informative for family members to get a general idea about what the therapy will look like and how it will progress but concise enough to allow the therapist to get right to the next step: forming an initial bond with each individual family member.

FORMING INITIAL BONDS

Forming a bond with each family member is essential to building strong therapeutic alliances, and strong alliances can mean the difference between whether a family stays in therapy or not, and whether treatment is successful.

Research has shown that the strength of the therapeutic alliance with parents predicts whether families complete treatment and that strong alliances with all family members predict better treatment outcome (Friedlander et al., 2011; Shelef et al., 2005). The therapist starts by getting a general sense of the fabric of each family member's life. They ask each family member a little about their work, studies, interests, extended family, and social network. However, because the session is only an hour long and there are many steps to traverse to establish relationship building as the shared goal of the treatment by the end of this first session, this initial exploration of each family member's life is necessarily brief. Practically speaking, the therapist typically asks each family member one or two questions about each domain just to become familiar with the broad strokes of their lives. Later, during parallel individual sessions alone with the young adult and parents separately, there will be more time to flesh out the details.

During this phase of the task, the therapist makes a conscious effort to highlight family members' competencies and strengths. For example, one father described his job as a high school principal. As he proudly conveyed the tremendous amount of responsibility his job entailed, the therapist made sure to acknowledge the father's accomplishments, skills, dedication, and how meaningful his work was. Such admiration and recognition, as long as it is genuine, are critical to forming a strong therapeutic bond with parents.

The parents we see often come to therapy feeling ashamed or like failures because their young adult is gay or transgender or because they themselves are struggling to accept their child. Acknowledging their accomplishments lets them know that we see them as more than just a parent who is conflicted, stuck, or having a hard time. Similarly, we listen for and acknowledge the young adult's strengths and competencies. For example, after one young adult described how she had been accepted to a prestigious internship at a top advertising firm, the therapist responded with admiration, noting how talented and hardworking she must be. By acknowledging young adults' strengths and competencies, we let them know that we see them as more than any struggles they may be having in their own life or in their relationships with their parents, and more than their sexual orientation or gender identity. It also reminds parents who have become overly focused on their young adult's sexual orientation or gender identity that their child is still the same, talented, unique, worthwhile, special person they were before they came out.

The therapist also pays attention to major stressors family members might be facing above and beyond parents' nonacceptance and the resulting rupture in the relationship. Parents sometimes report that they are struggling with health problems, dissatisfaction with their job, financial stress, or the burden of caring for their own parents. Young adults, on the other hand, are often grappling with normative developmental tasks, such as choosing a career path, supporting themselves financially, forming social bonds, and navigating romantic relationships.

In some cases, the young adult may be facing additional unique stressors, including discrimination at work or in other public spaces, victimization, mental health challenges, and substance abuse. The therapist briefly explores these various stressors in an empathic and supportive manner, taking such stressors into account when determining the pace and intensity of the therapy. For example, one family we (GMD, RBZ, and colleagues) worked with came to the first session shortly after one of the other children had been hospitalized following an epileptic seizure. The therapist was careful to allot time for parents to share their concerns about their younger child's recently diagnosed epilepsy and was as flexible as possible when scheduling sessions to accommodate medical appointments the parents needed to attend. The therapist's respect for, and sensitivity to, these parents' stress surrounding their other child's condition led to a stronger therapeutic bond and, ultimately, allowed the parents to commit to the treatment process with their young adult.

Asking about life stressors also provides an opportunity for the therapist to explore the extent of family members' support systems and coping strategies. The therapist asks both the young adult and their parents who they go to when they need a shoulder to lean on. Although some family members have extended family or good friends with whom they share their pain and fear, consult, and get support, others are more isolated and self-reliant. For those family members who have an intact support network, therapists later, in individual sessions, explore if and how they are using their network effectively, particularly in regard to stress and conflicts around the young adult's gender identity or sexual orientation.

For those family members who are more isolated, one goal of the therapy is to help them to identify and reach out to people in their lives who may be accepting and supportive—whether an uncle, coworker, or friend. In addition, the therapist may help family members access other available resources, including support groups; affirming members of the clergy; and, when indicated, mental health professionals. Many of the young adults therapists work with are either already in individual therapy when they present for ABFT-SGM or begin individual therapy during or after their work with us. In those instances in which family members are in concurrent individual therapy, we request that the family member give us permission to speak with their therapist in an effort to ensure synergy between the two treatments.

EXPLORING THE PRESENTING PROBLEM

Once the therapist has gotten to know each family member a bit and family members begin to feel more comfortable, the therapist turns to ask what brought them to therapy. Families come to us for various reasons and define the problem at hand in different ways. Often, it is the young adult who initiated the treatment and is the first to respond. The following example is taken from a first session with a young man, Tom,[1] who had been out to his parents for more than 5 years. Tom was 29, living independently, and clerking in a well-reputed law office. In the segment that follows, he describes to his parents how he has done his best to protect them by not coming out more publicly. At the same time, he conveys to them the price he has paid—and is still paying—because of not living openly and authentically. He states that the reason he has brought them to therapy is the hope that, by working together in treatment, he and they will be able to find a way to move forward together at an agreed on pace without his having to worry that they will fall apart emotionally, angrily blame him, or disconnect from him:

TOM: I know that the two of you wish that things would stay the way that they are now. But at some point, maybe not tomorrow but in the near future, I will be moving on with my life. I will have a partner, get married, and have children. I will post pictures on my Facebook page, and people are going to know—family, neighbors, friends. I want us to move on together, as a family, rather than have you feeling left behind or disrespected. I want to be able to share with you what is going on with me, in my life, without worrying it will cause you pain. I don't want to go back to that dark period when Dad stopped talking to me and you, Mom, sank into a kind of depression. I want us to move forward together.

In this segment, the young adult is assertive, clear, and compassionate. He is able to effectively articulate his coexisting needs for autonomy and relatedness.

In another case, a nonbinary client spoke about how it feels every time her parents misgender her (i.e., speak to her using the wrong pronouns). She described how invalidating and aversive such moments feel and how frustrated she is about what she perceives as her parents' lack of effort to understand and accept her for who she is despite their pronouncements of love and acceptance. She also spoke about the dysphoria she experiences

---

[1] All case examples have been disguised to protect client confidentiality.

when coerced to attend family events in typically male clothing, hide all information about her gender identity, and lie to family members she loves and believes would accept her if she were free to tell them the truth.

In yet another case, a young man shared his frustration and hurt resulting from the fact that, since coming out to his parents more than 2 years ago, they had not once mentioned his being gay or asked him about his personal life. He talked about how his parents were deeply and actively involved in both of his sisters' lives, often visiting them and their families or having them over for dinner but showed no interest in what was going on with him in his personal life, including whether he was alone or had a partner. He described feeling like his parents sacrificed having any type of meaningful relationship with him just because it is too hard for them to bear their disappointment and shame about his being gay.

The following example of the Cohen family illustrates the shift from the bond phase of this first task to talking about the presenting problem. This family consists of Natalie, a 27-year-old woman, her two parents who are both government workers, and three younger siblings. Natalie had come out to her parents as a lesbian 2 years earlier and was the one to initiate the treatment. The family is religious and lives in a tight-knit conservative community, which has made it harder for her parents to accept her sexual orientation. Over the years, Natalie has reported feeling increasingly unaccepted, isolated, and frustrated. Her parents' discomfort, disappointment, and fears have felt like a burden and both hurt and angered her. She and her parents have avoided conversation about her personal life. Moreover, her parents have not yet spoken to anybody about Natalie's sexual orientation, and they have made it clear that they expect Natalie to conceal her identity from her siblings, extended family, and others. The following segment occurred approximately 20 minutes into the first session with Natalie and her parents:

THERAPIST: So, Natalie, can you say something about what made you reach out to us at this time?

NATALIE: I wanted us to come because we don't talk.

THERAPIST: Can you say more?

NATALIE: Yes. (*Turns to her parents*) We aren't able to speak about certain issues. We can talk about my studies or my work, but there are things we still can't talk about—and any time we get close to those topics, things become tense, even explosive. In the end, I don't feel comfortable being at home. I know that it is difficult for the two of you to approach these issues as well—I think we can get help with this.

THERAPIST (*speaks to Natalie's parents, Sarah and Jacob*): Do you two also feel that way? That there are sensitive topics that you all can't talk about?

FATHER: Yes. And what happens is that, out of the blue, Natalie gets irritated. (*Speaks with a tone of anger and blame*) I feel like we are always walking on eggshells.

NATALIE (*becomes frustrated at being pathologized and blamed*): Of course it is like that! And it doesn't just come out of the blue or happen because I am moody. When you don't talk about things, they simmer under the surface, and all it takes is one cynical comment, and everything erupts.

THERAPIST: How long has it been this way?

NATALIE: It has always been this way. (*Turns to her parents and speaks in an accusatory tone*) I don't ever remember being able to tell you what is really going with me.

THERAPIST: Even when you were younger?

NATALIE: Yes, even when I was younger. And back then, I had nobody else to go to, either.

AMPLIFYING VULNERABLE EMOTIONS

At this point in the conversation, the therapist shifts the conversation away from family members' familiar feelings of frustration, anger, and helplessness and, instead, onto their underlying, more vulnerable emotions, such as fear, hurt, and loss. That is not to say that the young adult's anger at their parents for rejecting and hurting them is not legitimate, adaptive, and important to address. Quite the opposite. Later in the treatment, it will be critical for the young adult to fully connect with and express their adaptive assertive anger about being treated unfairly, set healthy boundaries, and clearly communicate their legitimate unmet needs. However, in these first moments of therapy, it is important to help the young adult begin from a place of vulnerability and longing. This is crucial for at least two reasons. First, helping the young adult access, explore, and express their adaptive but previously avoided vulnerable emotions helps them to form a more coherent narrative of their own experience and better understand and articulate their unmet needs. Second, the young adult's expression of pain and vulnerability usually elicits empathy in parents and activates their natural parenting instincts to care for; soothe; protect; and meet their child's legitimate, healthy needs.

Returning to the example of the Cohen family, to help Natalie connect with her more vulnerable emotions, the therapist invited her to recall a specific event or episode from the recent or more distant past in which she remembered feeling distressed and unable to share her feelings and needs with her mother and father. Activating episodic memories provides access to primary adaptive emotions and needs (Greenberg, 2011):

THERAPIST: Natalie, can you say more about that time when you were younger and felt like you had nobody to go to? What was going on?

NATALIE: I was in high school. I would come home, basically go up to my room, and cry all night from the evening until the next morning.

THERAPIST: What was going on inside you that was so painful at that time?

NATALIE: I was terrified (*begins to cry*). I felt like I was different from everybody else. I knew that there was something wrong with me. I prayed to God every night to make me normal.

THERAPIST: That sounds really lonely, really painful (*silence ensues*). And you felt like you couldn't say anything to your parents.

NATALIE: No (*begins to sob*).

These moments, when the young adult fully connects with and expresses their vulnerability, anguish, and loneliness in the presence of their parents, are both heart-wrenching and sacred. Often this is the first time that parents have witnessed their young adult's unadulterated pain. Such moments affect everybody in the room. Despite the parents' impulse to comfort their young adult or somehow alleviate their agony, it is essential that the therapist let such moments linger. Indeed, it is the young adult's pain that is the raison d'être and fuel for the treatment. The more powerfully it is felt, the more likely it is to elicit parents' empathy and motivation to better understand their young adult's feelings and needs and be there for them in a more attuned and responsive manner.

Once the young adult's pain is tangible in the room, the therapist turns to their parents to explore what it is like for them to see their child in such distress. Typically, parents are moved. They feel pain at witnessing their child's pain. In these moments, parents often become sad and tearful themselves, expressing sorrow and regret about their young adult's suffering. Their sorrow and regret are compounded by the fact that not only has their young adult suffered, but their young adult has been alone with that pain. At this moment, the job of the therapist is to keep parents connected to their sadness and regret and to amplify those feelings. The therapist does this not only to elicit parents' empathy and motivation to change but also because parents' expressions of empathic distress is a signal to their young adult that they have been heard and seen—and that they are cared about and not alone.

In this same case with the Cohen family, the therapist notices the mother, Sarah, beginning to tear up. She turns to Sarah directly:

THERAPIST: Sarah, you seem upset. Can you say something about what you are feeling right now?

MOTHER: It hurts me to see her hurting like that. She is my daughter. I love her. I want her to be happy.

THERAPIST (*speaks to both parents*): Did the two of you know that Natalie was suffering so during that period of time?

FATHER: No, we didn't know. She didn't say anything to us at all. We of course noticed that she didn't bring any friends home and spent most of her time in her room, but she insisted that she was fine, and she was excelling at school.

THERAPIST: What is it like now to hear her share how miserable she was during that period?

FATHER: It is upsetting. I had no idea she felt so bad (*voice begins to tremble*). It breaks my heart thinking what that must have been like for her.

MOTHER: It is horrible (*begins to tear up*). I feel terrible. It pains me to know that she was in such distress (*reaches over and gently rubs Natalie's leg*). I wish we would have known so that we could have supported her.

Again, it is important that such moments linger and sink in. The therapist must block parents' impulse to prematurely apologize or try to solve their child's pain or frustration (e.g., "I am sorry that we didn't see what was going on. How can we make it better?"). In these early moments, the goal is not to soothe the parents' distress or solve the young adult's problem. Our job as therapist is to hold parents steady as they witness, connect to, and validate their young adult's pain and unmet needs. The more fully parents connect to their young adult's pain, the more their natural, healthy instincts to care for and nurture their young adult are activated and the greater their motivation to use therapy to find a way to be there for their young adult in a more responsive, satisfying way.

DEALING WITH PARENTS' DEFENSIVENESS

In some instances, when parents witness their young adult's pain, they become defensive. Such defensiveness derives from their feeling guilty, blamed, or ashamed of having hurt or not supported their young adult. For example, at one point in the first session with the Cohen family, Natalie described having been startled and frightened by her mother's response to her initial coming out years earlier. Instead of validating Natalie's experience, her mother responded by disputing the accuracy of her daughter's narrative:

MOTHER: I don't think I yelled when you told me you were going out with a girl. Yes, I did tell you not to tell anybody else. I didn't want you to do anything that you might later regret. You have to understand. We were driving in a car, I was exhausted, and suddenly you asked me to pull over and then told me something that I was not prepared for.

During such moments, it is important for the therapist to immediately intervene. The therapist must first speak to the underlying, adaptive pain and regret the parent is experiencing seeing their young adult in pain. Second, the therapist needs to soothe the parent's feelings of shame, guilt, helplessness, and frustration. They must then redirect the conversation to the young adult's experience of feeling hurt, scared, unprotected, and alone. This sequence is illustrated in the following segment:

THERAPIST: Sarah, I can see by the tears in your eyes how much you love your daughter and how painful it must be to hear now how hurt, afraid, and alone she felt in that moment. I also hear that she shared this information with you at the end of the day, when you were exhausted, and that it was quite a shock. I know that you did the best you could in that moment. But it also sounds like your reaction scared and hurt your daughter.

MOTHER: Yes, I can understand that. I wish I could have responded differently.

Parents' sense of regret can be a powerful motivator to change as long as it is not overwhelming and does not turn into crippling self-criticism.

Parents' expressions of regret also signal to the young adult that something has shifted—that, perhaps for the first time, their parent recognizes how hurt they were, takes responsibility, and is open to hearing more.

In some instances, parents' defensive responses derive from the fear that they will be coerced into being more accepting or doing things that they do not agree with or feel ready to do. They mistakenly equate empathic listening and validation of their young adult's experience with the need to capitulate. They bristle at the idea of being browbeaten into compromising their values or lifestyle. As one father, Mr. Pine, said,

> I know that my son is unhappy. Maybe he is right to be disappointed or frustrated. I don't know. I know that he wants me to be more supportive, but I have to be honest: I don't think it is normal to be in a relationship with another man, and I am not going to act like I think it is or encourage him. He needs to understand that it is not easy for us. My wife hasn't stopped crying since he told us. If my father ever finds out, it will kill him. This has completely turned our lives upside down.

In the words of one mother,

> I know that she feels awful. It breaks my heart. I see her when she comes home for the weekend and goes up to her room. I try to get her to come down and be with everybody, but she just pushes me away. I wish it was different. I want her to be happy, to be a part of the family, but there is nothing I can do. She has two brothers who are about to take their college entry exams, and I don't want them to have to deal with this now. I feel like I am stuck in the middle.

This is a delicate moment in the therapy. It is critical at this point for the therapist to soothe parents by assuaging their fears that they will be judged or railroaded into changing their beliefs, or asked to do things that feel intolerable. Moreover, the therapist must maintain a posture of radical empathy with such parents, knowing that they feel trapped between their love for their young adult, on the one hand, and their belief system, culture, and social/family network, on the other hand. Parents may feel like their whole world is collapsing before their eyes. At the same time, the therapist needs to unequivocally validate the young adult's legitimate anger and pain and refocus parents' attention onto their young adult's suffering and unmet legitimate needs.

In the following segment from the earlier example of Mr. Pine, the therapist notices that Mr. Pine has become defensive, perhaps afraid that he is going to be forced to change in ways that he feels are impossible for him:

THERAPIST: Mr. Pine, I understand how you are feeling. This therapy is not about trying to make you change your beliefs or do anything you feel like you don't want to, or can't, do. I also hear loud and clear how hard this has been for you. When we meet alone next week, I want to hear more about what this whole process has been like for you and your wife, how you see things. We will also talk more about what you mean by acceptance. However, right now I see how pained your son is—feeling like he is a disappointment in your eyes, that he has lost your love and admiration, and that he feels disconnected from the family.

In most cases, once parents are assured that they will not be forced to compromise in ways that feel "wrong" or intolerable, they are able to reflect on and empathize with their young adult's pain and the effect that their nonacceptance has had on their young adult and on the relationship. In this particular case, once Mr. Pine's concerns were validated and he felt safer, he was able to at least momentarily see and connect with his young adult's pain and longing, lamenting, "Yes. I know how miserable he is. Believe me, I don't want to see him feeling that way."

EXPLORING THE RELATIONAL RUPTURE

Once the young adult's pain is palpable, the next phase of this task is to explore the dynamics behind the rupture in the young adult–parent relationship. The therapist invites family members to explore what has gotten in the way of the young adult's sharing with their parents their feelings about not feeling accepted and what has gotten in the way of parents' reaching out to their young adult in an effort to hear and understand their feelings and unmet needs. Young adults, for their part, are often hesitant to open up and share their vulnerable emotions because they anticipate being met with invalidating or even attacking responses from their parents. They would rather not be hurt, disappointed, or frustrated again. They may be afraid that their parents will argue with them about the facts (e.g., "That is not true. I don't treat your partner differently than I treat your sister's boyfriend") or minimize or invalidate their feelings and needs in a blaming, demeaning manner (e.g., "Nothing is ever going to make him happy unless we agree with everything he wants and says. He only thinks about himself"). Others anticipate that their parents will emotionally collapse or try to induce guilt (e.g., "It is too hard for me to think about. When I walk out of here, it is going to take me a week to recover").

Parents, for their part, avoid reaching out to their young adult because they are ambivalent, at best, about wanting to hear details about their young adult's life. That is because hearing about the details of their young adult's life experience makes their young adult's sexual orientation or gender identity tangible. This, in turn, evokes feelings of panic, fear, shame, guilt, grief, and helplessness. For example, hearing that their young adult is in a serious relationship and is, perhaps, planning to get married can not only shatter a parent's illusion that their young adult will eventually find a partner of the opposite sex and start a heteronormative family of their own but can also bring parents face to face with the possibility of having to attend their young adult's same-sex wedding. Likewise, hearing more details from their trans daughter about how she is discriminated against and harassed at her workplace can feel like a knife in parents' hearts.

In addition, at some level, parents are aware that the more they hear about, and empathize with, their young adult's pain and unmet needs, the harder it will be for them to continue with "business as usual." They know, whether consciously or subconsciously, that once they are fully connected to the emotional and psychological price their daughter is paying by having to conceal her identity from her grandparents, or that their son is paying by not being able to be with extended family on holidays, it will be harder for them to ignore or minimize their young adult's needs. They will be faced with the choice of either causing further emotional injury to their young adult or changing for their young adult's sake. The idea of making changes, such as coming out to their own parents or meeting their young adult's significant other, can be terrifying for parents. For all of these reasons, most parents we see are struggling between "wanting to know" and "not wanting to know."

The following segment from the Cohen family illustrates how the therapist explores the blocks in their relationship and what prevents family members from speaking more openly about the issues at hand:

THERAPIST (*speaks to Natalie*):   Do you know why you didn't say anything to your parents back then? Why you didn't go to them for comfort?

NATALIE (*turns to her mother*):   I was afraid of hurting you. I didn't know if you would be able to handle my distress. There have been times when I would tell you things that were bothering me, and it ended being all about you. I didn't feel like I had the energy to take care of you.

THERAPIST: And what about Dad?

NATALIE (*turns to her father*):   I didn't think you would want to hear. When I first mentioned that I thought that I liked girls, you told me not to talk about that, not to tell anybody—that it would pass.

THERAPIST (*speaks to Natalie's mother*): Did you know that Natalie was hesitant to share things with you because she was afraid that it might be too overwhelming for you to hear?

NATALIE: She has said this before. We have talked about this in bits and pieces. I feel like, because she knows that I had a difficult childhood and have been disappointed by my own family growing up, that she may feel the need to be a perfect child for me. . . . I am not fully sure where she gets this idea from—the feeling that she needs to make things perfect for me.

FATHER (*speaks to the therapist*): When Natalie told us that she liked girls 2 years ago, that was the first we heard about it. She just dropped it on us out of the blue. I was in shock. All I told her was not to tell others. We didn't know if it was a passing phase or if that is who she really was. We didn't want her to put herself in a position where she would jeopardize her future or be ostracized. Natalie has said a number of times that, in that moment, she lost all trust in us. That for her, that was a watershed event. We didn't fully understand that at the time. Now, it feels like she is angry with us all the time. We just try not to say things that might hurt her or lead to conflict.

NATALIE (*speaks to her father*): But even last year, you said that you would prefer that I not tell you if I had a girlfriend or about my activities working with the LGBT [lesbian, gay, bisexual, and transgender] community. You said that you didn't want to hear about those things. Maybe that has changed, but, if so, you haven't updated me.

FATHER: I admit that is not so easy for your mother and I to hear about those things. It is uncomfortable, something that we are struggling with.

OFFERING RELATIONSHIP BUILDING AS A SHARED GOAL FOR TREATMENT

At this point in the session, with family members more fully connected to their pain, the loss in their relationship, and their longing for things to be different, the therapist offers therapy as a way out of the relational impasse. The therapist presents the treatment as an opportunity for family members to create or recreate closer, more open, deeper, safer, loving, mutually respectful, meaningful relationships. Typically, the therapist will first turn to the young adult, as is illustrated in the case of the Cohen family:

THERAPIST: Natalie, I see how hurt you are by the way your parents have responded in the past and that you want them to know what it feels like when they make certain comments or ask you to hide who you are today. I also hear you saying that you wish things were different—that your relationship with them could be more open, less combative, and that they could be proud of you and not ashamed of your sexual orientation. If I could help you help them understand your feelings and needs, and respond in a way that felt validating and empathic, would that be something that would be worthwhile to you?

In most cases, the answer to this question is a resounding "yes." Such therapist statements give voice to, and validate, the young adult's adaptive hurt and anger and their deep longing to be heard, seen, respected, and embraced. It arouses hope—the possibility that this therapy will be a place where they will finally be understood by their parents.

NATALIE: Yes (*nods emphatically*). I think that . . . neither of them really understands how hard it is for me much of the time. I just want them to understand (*begins to cry*) and for us to be able to talk about things.

THERAPIST: Okay. That is what we are going to work on during this treatment.

To parents, the therapist presents the therapy as an opportunity for them to be there for their young adult in a way that they may not have been able to be there for them in the past. We offer therapy as a chance to build or rebuild a close, meaningful relationship with their child. In the following segment, the therapist reaches out to each parent in turn, speaking first to Natalie's mother, Sarah:

THERAPIST: Sarah, I see how much you love your daughter. I saw the pain in your face when she talked about feeling so hurt and alone. I see how torn you are. On the one hand, you want to be there to support her. On the other hand, you are anxious about having your family and friends find out that she is lesbian. If, however, somehow there was a way to help you feel less anxious, and you could be there for your daughter so that she could share her hurt and needs with you and so that she felt like you have her back, is that something you would like?

THERAPIST (*speaks to Natalie's father*): Jacob, I hear how difficult this is for you, how conflicted you are between your beliefs and your daughter's pain and needs. The two of you used to be so close, and that special bond seems to have been lost. If somehow it could be less difficult, less of a battle, and you were able to hear more about what was going in your daughter's life without it escalating into a confrontation about what is morally right or wrong, would that be something that you would want?

In most instances, the answer to these questions is, "Of course. That is why I am here. I want us to be a family again. We love our daughter and we want her to be happy, to feel like she is part of the family." That is why most families come to therapy. There is an inherent readiness and desire for change.

DEALING WITH RESISTANCE

In some cases, however, the young adult or their parents may be especially fearful or defensive. In these instances, therapists may have to work harder to create an environment that is sufficiently safe and trusting for family members to open up and agree to take a chance. To do this, we assure family members that we will adjust the pace of therapy according to their needs and abilities. We make it clear that we will not move forward faster than they, the family members, can tolerate. We assure them that they do not need to change their values and attitudes. We acknowledge that they may never see eye to eye and that the therapy may end up only being about creating safer and more mutually respectful relationships. We also encourage family members to let us know if they are feeling overwhelmed during the course of the session. We reassure them that throughout the treatment, we will protect them from hurting each other. We make it clear that the therapy room will be safe and that it is our job to make sure that they are heard and respected. All the while, we communicate hope and the expectation that family members will be able to transform their relationships in meaningful ways.

In the following example, a young man named Gal expresses doubt about his father's ability to really understand him and respond differently. He voices ambivalence about adopting relationship building as the goal for treatment out of fear of being disappointed and hurt once again:

GAL (*speaks to the therapist*): My dad grew up in a religious, homophobic family. I don't really have many expectations about him changing or of him becoming more accepting. There were times in the past when I thought that he had kind of gotten over it, and

> then suddenly he would become angry and tell me that I had
> to try harder to be straight. I am not sure that I want to put
> myself in that position again.

In that moment, the therapist worked to quell some of the young adult's
fears; create a sense of safety; and, at the same time, instill a sense of possibility that things might change as the result of the therapy:

THERAPIST: Gal, I hear you loud and clear. I am going to do my best to make
sure that nothing like that happens in the course of our work
together. Starting next week, I will be meeting with you and
your parents separately for a number of sessions. If I am not
convinced that you all are ready to talk together in a way that is
safe and productive, I won't put you in that position. With that
said, I have worked with many parents. Most have been able to
eventually listen better and respond better. Sometimes even a
little change can feel meaningful. Are you willing to give it a try?

In most instances, the young adult is willing to give it a chance, even if
they remain somewhat anxious or skeptical. In other cases, however, despite
the therapist's assurances, the young adult remains unconvinced that one
or both of their parents will be able to really understand. They feel too vulnerable to put themselves in the position to be disappointed or hurt again.
For example, one young woman responded to the therapist's question about
wanting a closer, more open and meaningful relationship with her parents
by saying,

> I think that at this point, I will settle for there being less tension in the relationship—to be able to come home for weekends and not worry about being
> insulted or that some comment will lead to a blowup.

At this stage of the therapy, with young adults who are expressing such fear
or hopelessness, this scaled-back goal is sufficient. It is an entrée. As the
work progresses and trust is built, family members often become increasingly hopeful and feel safe enough to allow themselves to believe and take
risks again.

WRAPPING UP THE FIRST TASK AND CREATING POSITIVE EXPECTANCY

At the end of this first task of the treatment, the therapist marks relationship building as the agreed on, shared goal of treatment. They echo family
members' longing for things to be different between them and offer therapy

as the path to reaching this goal. The following segment illustrates how the therapist concluded the first task with the Cohen family:

THERAPIST (*speaks to Natalie*):   Okay. That is what we are going to do here for the next few months. Natalie, I am going to help you help your parents understand some of the things you have gone through, how you are feeling now, and what will help you feel more connected and validated. (*Speaks to Natalie's parents*) Sarah and Jacob, I am going to help you two make sense of, and work through, some of your feelings about Natalie being a lesbian. I also want to help you feel less anxious, less stressed about reaching out to Natalie to hear and better understand what she has been through and what she needs in order to feel safe, understood, cared about, appreciated, and connected to you. Over the coming weeks, I will meet with Natalie alone and with the two of you alone for a number of sessions. Then, we will all get back together again to try to help you all talk about things that have been hard to talk about in the past. I want to help you all hear and respond to each other in a different way.

In ABFT-SGM, the therapist always ends the first task by engendering hope, regardless of how stuck the family is and how hard the road ahead appears to be. That is because in the great majority of cases we have treated, we have been able to help families make some progress, even when the beginning looks bleak or the ultimate outcome is far from optimal.

Therapists convey that we are experts and that we have lots of experience helping parents work through their fear, shame, grief, and internal conflicts and be more open, supportive, respectful, and validating of their young adult. We highlight any strengths we see in the family, such as their apparent love, care, and commitment to one another. The therapist will often say something like this:

I can see how much love there is in this family. I know you have been through a lot, but you are all here. I see how much you mean to one another. There are a lot of strengths in this family. I am very optimistic.

This first task of the treatment typically ends with families feeling like "we can do this together." Even in light of their fears and anxiety about not succeeding, they feel like they now have a direction and hope. Their love and care for each other is tangible as well as their mutual commitment to repairing their relationship. It is not uncommon for us to come out to the waiting room after this first session and find the family hugging each other, crying or walking out hand in hand.

4 ALLIANCE BUILDING WITH THE YOUNG ADULT

The second task in attachment-based family therapy for sexual and gender minority young adults and their nonaccepting parents (ABFT-SGM) is to build a strong working alliance with the young adult. This task is typically conducted over the course of three to six individual sessions alone with the young adult. The therapist begins by checking in with the young adult to see how they felt after the first session. Then, the therapist briefly explains the structure of the task. Next, the therapist turns their attention to getting to know the young adult as a person above and beyond their sexual orientation, gender identity, and relationships with their parents.

After forming an initial bond with the young adult, the therapist shifts to asking them about their experience of feeling rejected and unaccepted by their parents, and about the rupture in their relationship with their parents. The therapist helps the young adult to access and fully connect to their associated primary adaptive emotions (e.g., hurt, assertive anger) and unmet needs (e.g., the need to feel safe, to be prized, to feel like they belong). The therapist then explores the degree to which the young adult has (or has not) been able to convey these feelings and needs to their parents. The therapist

https://doi.org/10.1037/0000352-004

Attachment-Based Family Therapy for Sexual and Gender Minority Young Adults and Their Nonaccepting Parents, by G. M. Diamond and R. Boruchovitz-Zamir

FIGURE 4.1. Structure of the Alliance Building With the Young Adult Task

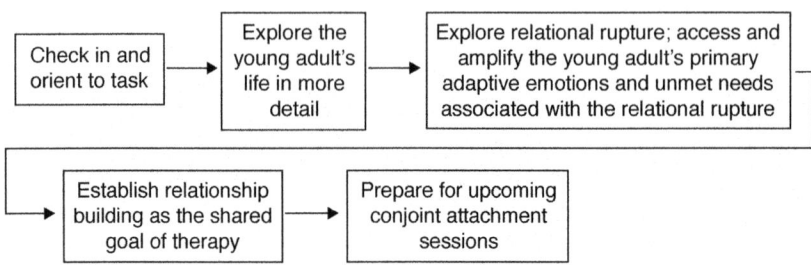

once again presents treatment as an opportunity for the young adult to feel more fully heard, acknowledged, understood, respected, and supported by their parents. Finally, the therapist prepares the young adult for subsequent conjoint attachment episodes (see Figure 4.1).

CHECKING IN

The therapist begins this task by checking in with the young adult regarding how they felt during and after the first session. Most young adults report feeling a sense of relief and guarded optimism. They typically describe having felt anxious before the first session, worried that their parents might be defensive and that emotions might escalate. However, in most cases, the first session goes better than the young adult had expected. In some ways, by the start of this second task, the young adult has already faced one of their biggest fears: sitting down with their parents in a room together and broaching some of the scary, difficult, and painful topics that had never been explicitly spoken about before—or at least not in the recent past.

The success of the first task elicits hope and motivation. Also, because of the clear structure of the treatment model and the empathy and skill of the therapist, the young adult typically feels like they are in good hands. They feel like the therapist understands their core pain, unmet needs, and fears. They see that the therapist is competent and has a plan. They also see that the therapist is assertive enough to protect both them and their parents from hurting each other.

In some cases, however, the young adult arrives for this second session still demoralized or skeptical—either because they were disappointed by their parents' responses in the first session or because they generally have little hope that things will change. These young adults may have already experienced

10,000 failed attempts to be heard, seen, validated, and treated respectfully. In such cases, the therapist acknowledges and normalizes the young adult's fear, frustration, and pessimism. At the same time, the therapist takes the position that this therapy will be different. They assure the young adult that they will be there to help and support them. The therapist makes it clear that it is their job to ready the young adult's parents so that they are more open and willing to listen. The therapist also expresses confidence in their ability to help the young adult's parents do better.

The following segments illustrate how therapists work to engage ambivalent young adults. First, the therapist empathizes with the young adult and validates their experience and frustration:

THERAPIST: I could see during the session last week how hard it was for you to get your parents to really hear how you feel when they make dismissive, disparaging comments. I saw that each time you began to share your feelings, they became defensive—that they were more focused on their own experience and needs than on how you felt.

Such empathy and validation can be powerful. The therapist was in the room with the young adult during the first session and witnessed their parents' difficulty in responding in an attuned, empathic manner. The young adult feels that *finally* somebody understands exactly what they are going through when they try to talk to their parents and why they are so frustrated. This shared experience creates a bond of understanding between the young adult and the therapist.

At the same time, the therapist is careful to highlight parents' expressions of love and their visible motivation and commitment to the process. These are reasons for hope, even if parents are not yet able to understand the effect of their rejecting words and behaviors. The therapist acknowledges that parents still have a long way to go and that one can never know how much they will change in the end:

THERAPIST: But I also could see how much they love you and how much they are willing to fight to make the relationship work, even if they don't yet know how to do that. I can't say for sure how this will play out in the end, but I am hopeful.

Finally, the therapist presents themselves as an ally. They are somebody who is experienced and skilled; somebody who knows how to work with parents to help them be softer, less defensive, more open, empathic, and reflective; and somebody who is also able to protect the young adult if and when their parents become critical, blaming, invalidating, or otherwise hurtful.

THERAPIST: I will spend a number of sessions working alone with your parents. I have a lot of experience helping parents be less defensive; to better hear their young adult and respond in a more open, reasonable, loving, respectful manner. However, if I am not confident that your parents can respond better, we won't get back together for conjoint sessions. I won't put you in that position.

Sometimes the therapist needs to be the one to hold the hope for family members until they, themselves, start to feel that things are beginning to change, and the benefits of the therapy begin to take their effect. For some family members, these first steps are a leap of faith.

GETTING TO KNOW THE YOUNG ADULT AND FORMING A THERAPEUTIC BOND

After checking in about the first session and, when necessary, restoring hope, the therapist begins exploring the contours of the young adult's life. The goal is to get to know the young adult as a person, beyond the reasons they have come to therapy. The atmosphere and pace of this phase of the task are more relaxed. It is just the young adult and therapist in the room, and there is a sense of spaciousness. The therapist typically begins this phase of the treatment by explicitly stating,

> Before we get into the reasons you came for therapy and what you would like to get out of the treatment, I want to take some time, now that we are alone, to better get to know you as a person.

The therapist then systematically explores the various domains of the young adult's life. They ask questions about work, studies, friends, hobbies/ interests, and romantic relationships. Because it is only the young adult in the room, the therapist can take more time and gather more details. Similar to the approach taken during the first task of treatment, the therapist pays careful attention to, and highlights, the young adult's strengths and accomplishments. For example, they might show interest in and admiration for the fact that the young adult is an accomplished pianist, was recently promoted at work, volunteers in a local youth group, or is an environmental activist.

The therapist's interest in the details of the young adult's life and focus on the young adult's strengths and accomplishments are important. It conveys that the therapist sees the young adult as an interesting, unique, multi-faceted, competent person—more than just their same-sex orientation, gender identity, or struggles with their parents. Taking time to get to know these other aspects of the young adult's life leads the young adult to feel cared about, soothes any fears they might have had about being pathologized or viewed singularly through the lens of their minority identity, and further facilitates the therapeutic bond.

EXPLORING STRESSORS IN THE YOUNG ADULT'S LIFE

Over the course of getting to know the young adult, being curious and excited about who they are as a person, and reveling in their accomplishments and successes, the therapist also pays attention to any major stressors the young adult may be dealing with above and beyond their parents' negative responses to their sexual orientation or gender identity. Sometimes young adults mention normative life challenges, such as being dissatisfied with their current job or trying to make ends meet financially. Sometimes they report unique challenges, such as struggling with anxiety, depression, or substance abuse; difficulties forming or maintaining positive meaningful social or romantic relationships; or coping with past traumatic events.

For many sexual and gender minority young adults, these challenges derive from, or are compounded by, *minority stress*—the stress associated with living in a stigmatizing, hostile, homo[trans]phobic culture (Meyer, 2003). Minority stress is the result of the prejudice, discrimination, and victimization lesbian, gay, bisexual, transgender, and queer (LGBTQ+) people regularly face in various domains of their life. This includes institutional discrimination, such as laws that restrict LGBTQ+ people's rights and access to basic services; prejudice in the workplace and in the community; and the hate, victimization, and microaggressions to which they are exposed in public and private spaces.

Such stress is not only detrimental in and of itself but can also lead to maladaptive stress responses, including rejection sensitivity, internalized homophobia (e.g., shame, self-hate), and attempts to conceal one's identity. These maladaptive stress responses, in turn, negatively affect the well-being of the individual and their functioning in the world (Hatzenbuehler et al., 2009). For example, the fear of being discriminated against at work can lead the young adult to invest great effort in concealing their identity. This may result in their avoiding contact with coworkers and having few or no close relationships in their workplace. That, in turn, can lead to a sense of isolation, loneliness, or even depression. Likewise, finding a romantic partner and forming a healthy intimate relationship can be complicated by the young adult's internalized stigma or rejection sensitivity.

Although extrafamilial stressors are not the foci of ABFT-SGM per se, they are important to explore during these individual sessions alone with the young adult for a number of reasons. First, when a young adult shares their distress, and therapists respond empathically, the young adult feels better understood, validated, and supported. This, in and of itself, can help to ameliorate loneliness, anxiety, and depression. It can also increase the level of trust and safety in the therapeutic relationship. Second, understanding the broader scope of what the young adult is up against as well as their coping strategies and internal resources is important information for the therapist as they calibrate the pace and intensity of the treatment. Third, in many cases, the young adult has never shared, or has stopped sharing, their stress, struggles, and associated emotions (e.g., fear, hurt, anger) with their parents. This is because of the rupture and lack of trust in the relationship as a result of parents' rejection of their minority identity. They may perceive their parents as uninterested or uncaring or may be afraid that their parents will judge them, minimize their struggles, blame them, use the information against them, lecture them, or prematurely try to problem solve.

This leaves the young adult unable to use their parents for support and guidance as they face various extrafamilial life stressors. This, in turn, places the young adult at greater risk for a variety of negative physical and mental health outcomes. Helping the young adult to articulate the intrapersonal and extrafamilial stressors and challenges they are facing and more fully connect to and express their associated vulnerable emotions and unmet needs prepares them to be better able to share some of these aspects of their lives in future in-session conversations with their parents.

Having young adults share their experience of intrapersonal or extra-familial stress and associated fear, hurt, shame, loneliness, and anger is important for two reasons. First, when parents witness—often for the first time—the depth of their young adult's suffering at work and in their personal lives, the challenges they are facing, and the injustices they deal with each day, their natural parenting instincts to support and protect their young adult are activated. Their assertive anger may lead them to advocate for their young adult in ways that they have not previously done. They are also motivated to support their young adult around these issues in subsequent conversations during conjoint attachment sessions. Second, understanding what their young adult is facing in their personal life drives parents to be more accepting and supportive as parents. They understand that their non-acceptance of their young adult's sexual orientation or gender identity is yet another source of disconfirmation and stress in their young adult's life. They become more motivated to be part of the solution rather than part of the problem.

In some cases, the therapist may recognize at this early stage of treatment that the young adult is coping with challenges that require interventions above and beyond the framework of ABFT-SGM. Such challenges include severe social anxiety, complex trauma, and substance abuse. These types of challenges typically require specialized, focused treatment. In such instances, the therapist may decide to refer the young adult for adjunct, concomitant individual therapy, medical consultation, or other resources.

EXPLORING THE YOUNG ADULT'S SUPPORT SYSTEM

In the next phase of this task, the therapist explores the extent and nature of the young adult's support system. They ask the young adult who they turn to for support when they feel alone, frustrated, scared, or down. Although many of the young adults whom ABFT-SGM therapists treat report having friends, a romantic partner, siblings, or other family members they can turn to, other young adults describe being isolated. This may be particularly true for young adults who live in rural areas or conservative communities and for young adults who are still actively concealing their identity from extended family, colleagues at work, or from past and current friends. As one young adult stated,

> I don't really have anybody to talk to. I have pulled away from most of my old high school and college friends. I told my sister that I am a lesbian, and she has pretty much cut off contact with me.

With young adults who are socially isolated, the therapist explores who in the young adult's social network may be a good but unutilized candidate to provide support. Many times, the young adult is able to identify a cousin, aunt, friend, or coworker they feel close to, who has been generally supportive in the past, and who feels safe. For example, one young adult considered the idea of opening up to one of their team members at work who was openly gay. They anticipated that this team member would respond in a supportive manner.

After assisting the young adult to identify potential sources of support, the therapist then helps them strategize regarding when and how to reach out to the chosen person. In some cases, the young adult may be hesitant. They may be embarrassed, ashamed, or afraid of being a burden or being rejected. In such instances, the therapist validates the young adult's anxiety and fear but, at the same time, reminds them of how alone they feel. The therapist emphasizes that everybody needs someone to lean on, somebody to share things with. That leaning on others is natural and adaptive. Finally, once the young adult has identified potential sources of support and has strategized regarding how to approach them, the therapist prepares the young adult to cope with potentially surprising, less than optimal responses from others.

EXPLORING THE YOUNG ADULT'S EXPERIENCE OF THEIR PARENTS' NEGATIVE RESPONSES TO THEIR MINORITY IDENTITY AND EXPLORING THE RELATIONAL RUPTURE

In the next phase of the task, the therapist shifts the focus to the reason the family has come for therapy: the young adult's experience of their parents' rejecting and nonaccepting responses to their sexual or gender identity and the effect of those responses on the relationship. Although some of this material was touched on in the first task, here the therapist seeks more detail. Because their parents are not present, the young adult does not have to worry about hurting their feelings, being attacked or invalidated, or having to defend themselves. They are freer to get in touch with feelings they do not usually express or might not even be aware of.

This is a core element of this second task of treatment. When young adults are more in touch with their emotions, they are able to form a more coherent narrative of what they went through in the past and may still be going through in the present. Their emotions also help them to clarify what they need now and in the future. Exploring these wounds, however, typically elicits painful emotions. The tone and intensity of the conversation change. For some young adults, this is the first time that they have connected with emotions other than anger and frustration.

In some cases, the young adult begins by describing acutely painful, even traumatic, memories surrounding their parents' responses to their coming out. For example, one woman described how her father had burst into her college dormitory in the middle of the afternoon and screamed at her after having seen a picture on Facebook of her at a party kissing a woman. She talked about feeling terrified by her father's rage and homophobic slurs. As she spoke, she began to tear up from a mixture of fear, hurt, and anger:

> He just stood there and screamed at me. He told me that I was never to see this girl again. I didn't know what he was capable of doing. From that time on, I realized that he was following me on social media. I had to find different ways to communicate with my friends and with my girlfriend. I was terrified.

Other young adults remember their parents responding to their disclosure by denying or otherwise invalidating their sexual orientation or gender identity. They describe their parents making comments such as, "You are just confused," "I know better than you who you are," "It is a passing phase," and

"You need to try harder—you just haven't found the right man." Some report that their parents accused them of being brainwashed by left-wing, progressive LGBTQ+ people, of being possessed or weak, or of taking the easy way out. Some report that their parents insisted that they seek counseling with either a religious authority or a therapist to help them "fix" their sexual orientation or gender identity and "get back on the straight and narrow path."

In other instances, young adults describe how their parents' initial positive, reassuring responses to their coming out waned over time, with their parents becoming less and less accepting. For example, one young adult recounted,

> What I remember was that both my father and my mother hugged me and told me that I was their son and that they would always love me. I could see, however, that they were quite in shock. It was a complete surprise for them— they had no idea. I was always into sports and had girlfriends. The way they responded and hugged me—that was important. But things started to change soon after. A few weeks later, I heard my father sobbing in his room. That was really hard. I had never heard him cry before. Then, over time, they began to fight. My father blamed my mother for being too soft with me. She, on the other hand, was angry at him for worrying more about what his own parents and siblings would think than about me.

Other young adults describe mixed responses to their coming out, with parents on one hand pronouncing their love and commitment to them but at the same time exhibiting fear and shame. For example, one young woman recounted her mother saying, "You are our daughter, and nothing will ever change that. In the meantime, however, do not tell anybody. You never know if, down the road, you will change your mind and then be sorry that you said anything."

In most cases, it is not only past wounds but also current, ongoing expressions of parental rejection and lack of acceptance that are causing the young adult distress and fueling the rupture in the relationship. For example, many young adults are hurt, frustrated, and angered by the fact that their parents are still unwilling or unable to hear about, or be positively involved in, their personal life. They describe how their parents refrain from asking questions about the day-to-day events of their lives, their friends, their romantic partners, and future plans, or how their parents disengage when they bring up such topics. As one young man described it,

> They never ask me about my personal life. They know nothing about my friends or work. I have been living in the apartment I am in for 3 years, and they have yet to come by to visit. If I tell them that I went up to the mountains for the weekend, that is the end of the conversation. They don't ask who I went with, if I had a good time. Nothing. You can feel that they don't want to know. They know nothing about my relationship with Avi or our thoughts about getting married and having a family in the future.

In many cases, parents' refusal to meet their young adult's romantic partner or include them in family functions is a central point of contention. One young man we (GMD, RBZ, and our colleagues) treated, who had been in a committed relationship and living with his partner for more than a year, reported that neither of his parents had met his partner despite his numerous invitations. His parents' response was always, "We don't feel comfortable. Perhaps when more time has gone by." The therapist explored how this young man's parents' refusal to meet his partner affected him and his relationship with them. He responded,

> It's hard. My partner, David, is so close with his parents, and we are over there all of the time—for holidays, weekends. I see what it could be like with my parents, but it is not. David can't really understand why my parents are the way they are. Those few times when I do go to my parents' house alone, without him, I feel like I am being asked to be somebody else, to hide part of me. Frankly, it is humiliating for both me and him. It's not fair. Sometimes, I find myself sitting at the dinner table alone with my two siblings and their partners. I am not willing to do that anymore. The irony is that if they were to meet David, I know that they would love him. If they are not able to change, I am afraid that I am going to see them less. They will be less a part of my life. We will end up growing apart. I don't want that, and I don't think that they do either.

Sometimes the rupture in the relationship is fueled by parents' repeated critical, demeaning, homophobic, or transphobic comments. For example, one young adult described how his father still mocks him each time he wears bright-colored socks, skinny jeans, or anything that does not adhere to traditional gender norms. He spoke about the pain and frustration he feels knowing that his father is embarrassed and ashamed about his being gay, particularly when out in public with him. Another young adult described the persistent, constant stress he experiences trying to make his voice sound deeper and control his mannerisms so as to appear less "feminine" when around his father.

Some young adults talk about the continued humiliation, loss, and frustration they experience as a result of being asked to conceal their identity from family members or others in the community. One young man's legitimate assertive anger was evident as he spoke about the price he is paying for respecting his parents' wishes that he not come out to his grandparents:

> I am tired of lying to my grandma and grandpa. I think they have a right to know, and it is important for me to have an open, honest relationship with them. We used to be close, and now I have to consciously avoid their questions about when I will find somebody or even what is going on in my life. I know that they will love me regardless.

Another young adult similarly talked about the tension between them and their parents around coming out as nonbinary to extended family:

> I am not willing to hide who I am anymore. My parents are concerned about how others will react and whether certain branches of the family will shun us or me. I am not worried about that. Whoever is accepting will be accepting. Those who are not—that is their problem. I am at peace with who I am. This has been a point of contention between me and my parents. They are so afraid about what others—especially their own parents—will think.

Other young adults report that their parents still cast doubt on the authenticity of their sexual or gender identity, even years after their coming out. As one genderqueer young adult described, "My parents think that if I would spend less time with LGBTQ+ friends and reconnect with my old friends, everything would go back to the way it once was." Another young woman described how her mother outright tells her that she knows who she is and what her sexual orientation is better than she herself knows. She described how her mother tells her she is straight and just confused.

Indeed, many young adults report that their parents continue to harbor hope that one day, they will identify as heterosexual or cisgender even though, at some level, their parents know that this is likely not the case. They describe how their parents still ask them about former other-sex, cisgender romantic partners; encourage them to try dating people of the other sex; call them by their birth names and assigned gender pronouns rather than their chosen name and pronouns; leave them articles about those who have "successfully" undergone sexual orientation change "therapy" or "counseling"; and convey their disappointment and grief about their identity in a manner that is meant to induce guilt and feels coercive.

Yet other young adults describe their primary concern as one of boundaries and respect for who they are as a person. As one young woman described it,

> I am not willing to sit around the dinner table and hear my relatives make homophobic comments. That is me that they are talking about and my community. I expect my father to say something—to put his siblings in their place. When I get angry and stand up for myself or others, they accuse me of overreacting— making a big deal of nothing. I have had to put up with that my whole life, and I am not willing to be in that position anymore. I am going to say my mind whether they like it or not.

ACCESSING AND AMPLIFYING PRIMARY EMOTIONS

Many of the young adults therapists see are initially more in touch with their frustration and anger about their parents' nonacceptance than they are with their underlying vulnerable emotions, such as hurt, fear, shame, and grief.

This is understandable. Vulnerable emotions are threatening. Being vulnerable in the face of invalidating, critical parents can feel dangerous. Rejecting anger, on the other hand, feels empowering. When on the attack, one feels more in control. Rejecting anger, however, is what Greenberg and colleagues have termed a *secondary emotion* (Greenberg & Pascual-Leone, 2006). It is a secondary, defensive response to the immediate, primary, natural, and adaptive feelings of hurt and fear one experiences when emotionally injured or threatened. Although such defensive responses can feel good or protective in the short run, in the long run, rejecting anger both makes the young adult feel worse about themselves and pushes their parents away, leaving the young adult feeling even more alone and disconnected. Secondary emotions also obscure underlying primary adaptive emotions that help the young adult make sense of their experience and needs. For that reason, secondary emotions are, by definition, maladaptive.

Accessing one's underlying primary adaptive vulnerable emotions, on the other hand, is important for a number of reasons. First, when the young adult is aware of their hurt, fear, shame, and grief, they have a better, more complete understanding of what is going on inside them and why they are responding in the manner that they are.

Second, access to our primary adaptive emotions informs us of what we need (Greenberg, 2012). For example, when we are hurt by somebody, we need to know that they recognize that they have hurt us, take responsibility, show regret, and commit to treating us better the next time. When sad or alone, we need others to reach out to us, hug us, and offer support. When ashamed, we need others to remind us that we are valuable.

Third, and central to ABFT-SGM, when young adults are aware of and connected to their vulnerable emotions, they are better able to express them directly to their parents in subsequent conjoint attachment sessions. Research has shown that expressing vulnerability facilitates relational repair (McKinnon & Greenberg, 2017). When young adults convey their pain, vulnerability, and their need to be understood, comforted, supported, recognized, or protected, parents are more likely to be empathic and respond in kind. The young adult's vulnerable emotions elicit in parents the urge to soothe and protect them and better meet their needs. In contrast, when young adults criticize, blame, or attack their parents, their parents are more likely to withdraw or retaliate, exacerbating the rift in the relationship. For that reason, at this phase in the task, the therapist aims to amplify the young adult's vulnerability. Later in the task, the therapist also helps the young adult to process their legitimate adaptive anger at being violated and prepares them to express this anger and set boundaries with their parents in a clear, regulated, effective manner.

In the following example, the therapist begins by validating the young adult's legitimate assertive anger at her parents for disconnecting from her and excluding her from the family. As the conversation continues, however, the therapist gradually explores previously avoided but core vulnerable emotions and unmet needs. The young adult, Sharon, is a 28-year-old religious woman who had come out to her parents 4 years earlier. She was living on her own in another part of Israel and only periodically went home to visit her family for the weekend. She spoke angrily about how her parents demanded that she keep her sexual orientation a secret. They explicitly told her that she was compromising their standing in the community. They also did not want her to influence her younger siblings:

SHARON: They make me feel that there is something terribly wrong with me, like I am some kind of monster—that it would be better if I was dead or would have never been born. That is not what parents are supposed to do. They are supposed to make their kids feel good about themselves, like they are a part of the family. It makes me so angry. That is why I usually stay in my apartment alone on weekends rather than come home.

THERAPIST: I can understand why you would be angry. That sounds horribly unfair. I can also imagine you in your apartment all by yourself and how alone that must feel.

SHARON (*begins to cry*): Yes, it is horrible. My friends are all at their parents' homes on the weekend. I am completely alone, and I don't think my parents really care. I really have nobody.

THERAPIST: That sounds terrible. That must really hurt. (*A long silence ensues.*) I am so sorry. (*Sharon begins to sob.*) Can you say what you need from them in those moments, what would help you to feel better?

SHARON: Yes. I expect them to call me and ask me how I am doing. I expect them to invite me on Fridays. I can always decide whether I want to come or not, but I want to feel like I am wanted, that I have a place in the home. Like they are there for me.

Helping the young adult to more fully connect to their hurt, loss, grief, loneliness, and longing is no fun. In these moments, young adults often experience intense pain accompanied by uncontrollable sobbing. Such episodes can be extremely hard and scary for the young adult, who may not be used to such strong affect and the accompanying sense of loss of control. These moments can also be hard for therapists, who themselves may feel uncomfortable or shaken by the young adult's intense pain. Therapists may fear that they are eliciting too much or unnecessary pain and be concerned that the young adult will be overwhelmed, collapse, and be unable to pull themselves out of it.

In these moments, the therapist must lean into these feelings. We must help the young adult fully connect to, and express, their previously avoided but adaptive emotions and unmet existential needs, no matter how painful they are. Unprocessed traumatic memories and disavowed repressed or thwarted emotions deriving from parents' rejection continue to affect not only the welfare of the young adult but also the quality of the young adult–parent relationship—even years later. They are like seething wounds breeding anxiety, fear, and resentment. They drive the young adult's maladaptive responses, including avoidance, self-criticism, and aggression. Lancing and working through these emotional wounds and helping the young adult to better articulate their underlying emotions and adaptive needs are an essential first step in preparing the young adult for more productive interactions with their parents in subsequent conjoint attachment sessions.

ESTABLISHING RELATIONSHIP BUILDING AS THE SHARED GOAL OF THERAPY

Once the young adult's underlying pain and fear have surfaced and their unmet needs clarified, the therapist again turns their attention to the relational rupture and their longing for connection. They do this by asking the young adult if they have ever shared these feelings and needs directly with their parents. This is the same intervention that was introduced in the first task of the treatment, during the initial conjoint session. However, now, after all of the work that has been done throughout this second task, the young adult has a much deeper, clearer, more coherent narrative of their story. Their emotions are now anchored in meaning. They are more connected to, and able to fully articulate, their pain, fear, assertive anger, and unmet needs. They also are more accepting of their emotions and needs, seeing them as real and legitimate. They feel more justified in asserting themselves and more deserving of being understood and treated with care and respect. At this moment, when the young adult is most connected with their adaptive emotions and legitimate unmet needs, the therapist again offers therapy as an opportunity for the young adult to be more fully heard.

Returning to the case example of Tom first presented in Chapter 3, in the following segment, the therapist reintroduces the goal of relationship building. Earlier in the task, Tom had described having once been very close to both of his parents and a great source of pride for them. However, since his coming out, his relationship with his parents had deteriorated. His parents blamed him for causing the family to fall apart and were uninterested in his feelings and needs. In the following segment, the therapist first marks and validates Tom's pain and frustration and then presents the upcoming attachment task as an opportunity for him to finally feel heard and understood:

THERAPIST: You know, Tom, it comes through so clearly how painful that whole period was for you, just after you came out. I wonder if your parents know how hard that time was for you.

TOM: My impression, based on talks I have had with them, is that they don't really want to remember. When I attempted to bring it up in the past, they tried to wrap it up and sweep it under the table with sentences like, "That was a difficult period for us. We were in crisis mode," without really wanting to understand what it was like for me. Some of the things they even denied ever happened. They just want to put a lid on it and move on. But that doesn't work. That is what led to the explosion and cutoff from my father the last time.

THERAPIST: So, it is hard for them to really hear what things were like for you.

TOM: Yes, despite the fact that I wrote everything in detail in the letter that I gave them. What it was like for me, the difficulties, the pain, the struggle during that period between the ages of 13 and 21 before I came out to them.

THERAPIST: Is that something you would want them to understand more?

TOM: Absolutely. That is part of the process I have gone through. It is not like, one morning, I woke up and thought to myself, "How exciting—I like boys" (*smiles cynically*). It's a process that accompanied me for a long, long time and impacted me greatly. And it's things that they didn't know about their son. They didn't know what was going on with me at school, they didn't know what was going on with me at night, what was going on with me and my friends, what was going on with me inside!

THERAPIST: Okay. That is what I would like to help you do when we all meet together next week. I want to help you share some of your experiences with them, help them understand what things have been like for you. How does that sound to you?

TOM: That is exactly what I am hoping for—for them to finally hear what it has been like for me and what it is still like for me.

Although Tom is enthusiastic about finally being able to share his experience with his parents, for many young adults, the idea of speaking directly to their parents about feeling disappointed, hurt, and angry arouses anxiety. These young adults may fear how their parents will react. They may be concerned that the potential cost or backlash from such conversations outweighs the potential benefits. They may also fear being overly vulnerable and hurt, losing control, or shutting down.

In the following example, Maya, a 27-year-old bisexual woman, describes how throughout the first few weeks of the therapy, her parents had made tangible steps to improve their relationship with her and that, now, she is afraid of "rocking the boat." She expresses her concern that talking with them about past injuries might, at this point, be counterproductive:

MAYA: Things have been good this week. I went to the beach with my sister and my father and had a great time. The next day, he asked me to send him a picture of me and my girlfriend. Which brings me to the topic that I wanted to talk about: I am scared to death that by getting into things from the past, I will go and ruin the whole thing, all of the gains we have made.

THERAPIST: Can you say more?

MAYA: I know that talking about things from the past is important. I am just afraid that they will interpret it as me not appreciating the progress they have made or that it will make them feel guilty. Also, I have just recently learned how to express anger. I am afraid that a conversation about the past will elicit those parts of me.

THERAPIST: And what is scary about that?

MAYA: That they, my parents, will be angry with me in return. That it will get out of control.

At this point, the job of the therapist is to acknowledge the young adult's fears and ambivalence; amplify their longing to be heard; remind them that their parents have chosen to come to the therapy and are committed to the process; and assure them that they, the therapist, will be there to help if they or their parents become upset or defensive.

THERAPIST: Maya, I can understand your concerns. This is new and scary territory. However, based on conversations I have had with your parents over the past few weeks, I don't think your opening up to them is going to ruin things or chase them away. Your parents are here for a reason. They know what we are doing here—it is not a secret. They are here because they, too, want to have a closer, more open, honest relationship with you. I think that they want to hear what you have to say as much as you want to say it. In any event, I will be there in the room with you, and if I feel like things are escalating or that your parents are having a hard time, I will intervene to help them.

MAYA: I don't want to cause them pain or ruin things.

THERAPIST: Your parents have said that what is most important for them is repairing the relationship, even if it involves hearing difficult things along the way.

PREPARING FOR THE UPCOMING CONJOINT ATTACHMENT TASK

Once the young adult is signed on to the goals of the upcoming attachment task, the therapist shifts to the next and final phase of this task: preparing the young adult for upcoming in-session conversations with their parents. Such preparation is important because it increases the likelihood that these conversations will go well. Family members are not used to engaging in sustained conversations about difficult, painful topics. Their natural instinct is to avoid such conversations, either by premature problem solving, distraction, or changing the topic. For future in-session conversations between the young adult and their parents to be meaningful, potent, and productive, the content, affect, and process all need to be right.

Good content touches on core attachment- or identity-related themes. These themes include the young adult's feeling rejected, abandoned, betrayed, unprotected, excluded, alone, not understood, invalidated, unloved, or like a burden. It is these core experiences that fuel the young adult's anxiety, pain, or anger. These topics need to be at the center of the conversation. In contrast, conversations focusing on the manifest, superficial details of the latest argument (i.e., who did what to who) are unproductive. Such conversations tend to go in circles and escalate rather than getting to the root of the young adult's core experience and unmet needs. Not all content is created equal. For this reason, the therapist helps the young adult choose two or three core themes that are important for them to bring up with their parents during the upcoming attachment task so that this material is easily available when the time comes.

Just as the content of future attachment sessions needs to be right, so does the affect. As mentioned earlier, when young adults begin by expressing rejecting, blaming anger toward their parents, parents are likely to become defensive and shut down. In contrast, when the young adult is able to begin such conversations by expressing hurt, shame, loneliness, and fear and disclose their unmet needs from a place of vulnerability rather than in a demanding, blaming fashion, parents are more likely to listen and respond with empathy and support. This does not mean that the young adult's assertive anger is not important. Quite the opposite. We (GMD, RBZ, and our colleagues) have simply found that parents are more likely to engage in this process when their young adult starts from a place of vulnerability and need.

When possible, the therapist helps the young adult to identify paradigmatic instances or events—episodic memories—to share with their parents during upcoming in-session conversations. This is important because accessing episodic memories helps the young adult's experience come alive and allows parents to relate better. Episodic memories activate all aspects of the young adult's emotion schema, including their physiological arousal and action tendencies, which are then expressed in a visible, tangible manner. For example, when fully connected, a young adult's grief will be evident by their facial and bodily expressions, and their sobbing. During such moments, their unmet need to be comforted and soothed is undeniable.

Finally, the therapist addresses any concerns the young adult might have about how the process of upcoming conversations with their parents will unfold. Some young adults are afraid that they will not know how to start. Others are afraid that the moment that their parent responds in their typical dismissive or hurtful manner, they will become frustrated or lose their motivation and give up. Yet others worry that things will escalate and blow up. To avoid such pitfalls, the therapist takes time to go through each of these scenarios and helps the young adult plan for each eventuality.

As part of the preparation, the therapist asks the young adult ahead of time for permission to remind them what they had decided to talk about if they see them getting stuck during the attachment sessions. They also speak with the young adult about realistic expectations and the possibility of initially suboptimal parental responses. Indeed, the therapist suggests that this is inevitable. They predict that the responses of the young adult's parent will not be perfect the first or second time they try. Old habits die hard. The therapist encourages the young adult to be patient and to persevere, rather than get frustrated, withdraw, or lash out. They remind the young adult that they will be there to gently but firmly redirect their parents and that such conversations are a matter of successive approximation. Two steps forward, one step backward; as long as the conversation is moving in the right direction, the process is good. The therapist assures the young adult that if they see that the conversation is escalating, they will intervene, that they are there to make sure that family members do not hurt one another and that the therapy room remains a safe space.

By the end of this task, the young adult should be signed on to the goals for the upcoming conjoint attachment sessions, feel prepared, and feel optimistic about their success. The therapist reminds the young adult that they have been meeting separately with their parents over the past few weeks to get them prepared. We assure them we will not initiate conjoint sessions until we feel that their parents are ready and able to respond to their feelings and needs in a more open, caring, and validating manner. Young adults typically finish this task cautiously optimistic—hopeful that things can be different.

5 ALLIANCE BUILDING WITH PARENTS

The third task of attachment-based family therapy for sexual and gender minority young adults and their nonaccepting parents (ABFT-SGM) is to build strong working alliances with parents. This task is conducted over the course of several sessions with the parents together or, if needed, with each parent alone—without the young adult being present. The therapist begins by checking in with each parent to see how they felt after the first session. Then, the therapist turns their attention to getting to know each parent as an individual, above and beyond the reasons they have come for treatment. This phase of the task includes exploring parents' strengths and the stressors they are facing in their lives, their support network, and each parent's own attachment history. Next, the therapist invites parents to share what it has been like for them to have a sexual or gender minority young adult. The therapist then invites parents to reflect on how their difficulty accepting their young adult's identity has affected their young adult and their relationship with them. Once parents begin to reflect on and empathically connect to their young adult's pain and unmet needs, the therapist presents treatment as an opportunity for parents to be there for their young

https://doi.org/10.1037/0000352-005
Attachment-Based Family Therapy for Sexual and Gender Minority Young Adults and Their Nonaccepting Parents, by G. M. Diamond and R. Boruchovitz-Zamir

FIGURE 5.1. Structure of the Alliance Building With Parents Task

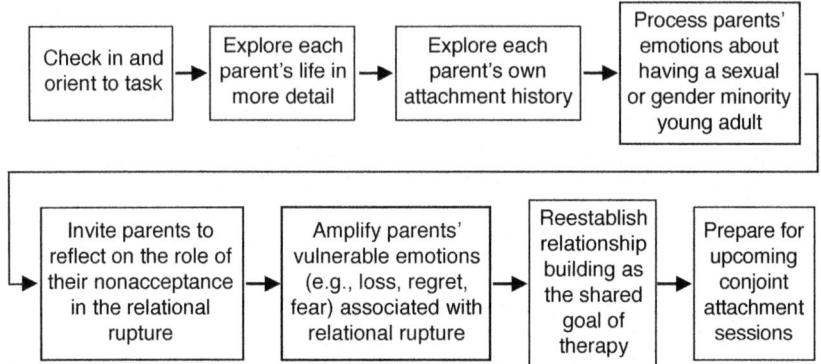

adult in a more responsive, validating, and supportive manner. Finally, the therapist prepares parents to reach out to, and be there for, their young adult in subsequent conjoint attachment sessions (see Figure 5.1).

CHECKING IN

The therapist begins this task by checking in with parents regarding how they are feeling after the first session. For many, it was the first time they had ever heard their young adult speak openly about their experience of being lesbian, gay, bisexual, transgender, and queer (LGBTQ+) and their feeling of being unaccepted, unsafe, disappointed, hurt, and alone in the family. This can be a painful experience for parents and can elicit feelings of remorse. These feelings may still be lingering when parents come for their first session alone with the therapist.

The following example is from the first session alone with David and Eileen Levy, the parents of Alex, a 30-year-old gay man and mechanical engineer who lives with his partner in the same city as his parents. Five years before, Alex's parents had inadvertently found out that he was gay. Ever since, there has been no conversation between Alex and his parents about his being gay. Although he and his parents have been in contact multiple times a week and spoken about day-to-day matters, all have avoided talking about anything related to his sexual orientation. Alex's parents have been avoidant because the topic causes them distress. Alex has avoided the topic because he is afraid of hurting his parents and of being disappointed by their responses. In the following excerpt, Alex's father, David, describes how he felt after the first session and hearing his son speak for the first time about the intense shame, fear, and alienation he had experienced during his teenage years:

FATHER: It was hard to hear some of the things Alex said. When I look back, I try to see where I made mistakes, didn't see things, or protect him enough. I remember that one day, he came to me and told me that some of his friends from school had distanced themselves from him, stopped inviting him to join them in various activities. I didn't see it. I didn't pick up on the cues. Hearing him talk last week, I realized that we, Eileen and myself, have been avoiding things, signals, his whole life, and that it has impacted him.

In such moments, when parents are feeling sad, guilty, self-critical, and ashamed, the therapist responds with compassion and encourages parents to be compassionate toward themselves. Some level of remorse is a good thing. It serves to motivate parents to do better. Too much remorse, however, can lead to paralyzing rumination and self-criticism. Thus, in these moments, the therapist validates and normalizes parents' feelings of regret and guilt. The therapist reflects to them that they did the best they could at the time. They also affirm the parents' love and concern for their young adult's welfare and remind the parents that this therapy is a chance for them to be there for their young adult in a more responsive manner—in a way that they perhaps wished they could have been there for them in the past.

Although most parents leave the first session feeling some degree of remorse, other parents are more defensive. They may have felt blamed, judged, or unappreciated by their young adult during the initial session and, in turn, left the session frustrated and annoyed. Now, alone with the therapist, they are often anxious to share "their side of the story" and "let off steam." They may dispute the historical facts as told by their young adult or blame their young adult for being too sensitive, too demanding, or unwilling to do their part to fix the relationship. Returning to the case example of the Cohen family first introduced in Chapter 3, such defensiveness is evident in the following example from the first session alone with Natalie's parents:

FATHER: I was quite shocked by some of the things that Natalie said last week. Some of it was simply not true. When she said that we asked her to not say anything to anybody, that was in the days immediately following her telling us that she was attracted to women. Since then, we have never told her who to tell and who not to tell. I have no problem with her telling whoever she wants. Part of the tragedy with Natalie is that in the past couple of years, we haven't had a close relationship with her, and she didn't share her pain, and so we couldn't be there for her.

Natalie's mother, clearly distressed, continued:

MOTHER: We actually went out of our way to make Natalie feel comfortable despite it being hard for us! When I see her come home sad or irritable, I go to her room, try to speak with her, encourage her to come be with us in the living room instead of holed up in her own room with the door closed, but she shuts me out. She is the one who pushes us away. It is not for a lack of our trying to talk to her.

In such instances, the therapist acts to soothe parents' concerns about being blamed or judged; acknowledges their love and commitment to their child; and empathizes with their frustration that despite their best intentions and efforts, something is still undermining the relationship. The therapist reiterates that the work of therapy will be to help them better understand what is fueling their young adult's hurt, anger, and avoidance and how to better position themselves to help their young adult feel heard and recognized. In this particular example, the therapist responded in this way:

THERAPIST: I can see how frustrating this is for you both. I see how much you love your daughter and care about her. You have worked so hard to do your best despite feeling conflicted about her sexuality. Yet, somehow, something is still getting in the way, like she needs something different. I understand that not everything she wants is possible, but I want to help you try to figure out what she needs to feel safe enough to open up, feel understood, and feel accepted. I am going to help you with this. That is part of what we are going to do in this therapy.

GETTING TO KNOW EACH PARENT AND FORMING THERAPEUTIC BONDS

After checking in regarding their experience of the first session, the therapist moves on to deepening their bond with each parent. Such bonds are critical because much will be asked from parents over the course of the treatment. If parents do not feel like the therapist knows them, respects them, and understands their point of view and the stressors in their life, they will be less likely to trust and rely on the therapist when things become challenging. This process of building therapeutic bonds begins with the therapist's taking time to get to know each parent as a person, beyond the reasons that have brought them to therapy.

The atmosphere and pace of this phase of the task are more relaxed. The therapist typically begins by explicitly saying that they want to take some time to get to know each parent and then asks each of them to share a little about themselves, including where they work, what they like to do for enjoyment, and who is in their current family and friend network. The therapist also asks about any stressors parents are dealing with above and beyond their difficulty accepting their young adult's sexual or gender identity.

The parents we (GMD, RBZ, and our colleagues) see come from all walks of life. Some are airline pilots, university professors, teachers, or police officers. Some own their own business or work in retail or factory jobs. Some are retired and some are unemployed. They also have diverse interests. For example, some we have seen enjoy sports and exercise; one was member of an amateur dance company, and another restored antique furniture as a hobby. In terms of their social networks, some parents have described having a robust and long-standing network of close friends who have been together since, or even before, their children were born. They have been fixtures in each other's lives throughout the years, participating in each other's major life events. Others have described being more isolated—having few close friends or, in some cases, no close friends at all.

Parents also vary greatly in terms of their extended family network. Some lost their parents when they were young; others have had frequent meaningful contact with their parents, who still play an active, key, and positive role in their lives. Some parents have reported little or no contact with their siblings. Others have described being close to their siblings and attending regular gatherings with extended family.

In terms of stressors, some parents are dealing with physical or mental health issues; others are anxious about making ends meet financially. Some parents are caring for an elderly parent; others are dealing with stressful situations at work. Most parents also have had other children aside from their young adult who is participating in the therapy. Each of these other children can present their own set of concerns and challenges for parents.

Throughout this process of getting to know the fabric of each parent's life, the therapist listens for, and highlights, strengths, resources, and accomplishments. Parents typically begin this treatment feeling vulnerable and ashamed, so our recognizing their strengths and competencies serves to create safety and trust. At the same time, we express empathy and support when parents talk about their losses or the challenges they are facing.

EXPLORING PARENTS' SUPPORT SYSTEMS

In the next phase of this task, the therapist segues into exploring who parents turn to in times of distress and need. Identifying sources of social support may be particularly important for parents participating in ABFT-SGM. Such parents often present for treatment with high levels of shame, fear, sense of loss, and global distress about their young adult's sexual or gender identity. Many of the parents we see have been alone with these feelings for years—ever since their young adult's coming out. In some cases, they have not shared their secret with anyone at all.

Positive, accepting responses from close others can mitigate parents' shame and fear that they will be negatively judged, pitied, or ostracized. Such support and positive reactions from others can help normalize their young adult's sexual or gender minority identity for them. Parents who disclose their young adult's identity to close friends, family, and others, and share their feelings, report relief and greater well-being. Indeed, findings from qualitative studies suggest that acceptance and support from family and friends are determining factors in parents' own acceptance process (Saltzburg, 2004). Importantly, when parents themselves are in less distress, they are more psychologically available to hear, reflect on, and respond productively to their young adult's experience of feeling not accepted and to their young adult's unmet attachment and identity needs.

Those parents suffering from high levels of shame and fear tend to be those who most try to conceal their child's identity. They withdraw from social interactions. Ironically, this leaves them even less likely to receive the family and social support they so need. Some fear that disclosing their young adult's minority identity will lead their family to be seen as less "perfect" or themselves to be seen as failures as parents. Other parents are afraid of making their friends and extended family feel uncomfortable or burdened.

To combat parents' shame, fear, and avoidance and help them better use their family and social networks, ABFT-SGM therapists highlight and amplify the tremendous psychological and emotional price that they and their young adult are paying because of their secrecy and hiding. We help parents connect with their adaptive but unmet need for support, comfort, and validation from others. We also work with parents to identify opportunities for them to disclose to more people. This typically involves helping parents think about who among their family members, friends, and colleagues at work are most likely to respond in an accepting, or at least supportive, manner.

We might then help parents plan how and when to reach out to these people, how to garner the courage to take this scary step, and how to cope with potentially disappointing or negative responses. We also refer parents, when indicated, to LGBTQ1 affirmative parent support groups in the community, such as PFLAG.

The following example is drawn from an alliance-building session with Alex's parents, David and Eileen. In the segment that follows, the therapist explores Alex's parents' readiness to share their distress with family and friends and use them for support. As often happens, each parent was in a different spot in terms of their level of acceptance and readiness to disclose. Alex's mother described being concerned about burdening her own mother and siblings and causing them unnecessary pain. In contrast, Alex's father had seemingly reached a point at which he was ready to assert himself, regardless of the consequences. He stated that he was no longer willing to hide his son's sexual orientation. He was fed up with feeling ashamed and felt like his son deserved an ally and advocate:

THERAPIST (*speaks to mother*):   Do people in your family share personal stuff with one another when they are in distress? When life's challenges rear their heads?

MOTHER: We don't talk about things that are upsetting. People in our family mostly talk about things that are going well. Sometimes we share things when we are upset, but we choose carefully when and how much to share such things.

FATHER: My wife's mother is the one who centralizes all of the information. She is the "dispatcher." She is careful to relay the information in measure. She titrates the information to make sure that nobody gets too upset.

THERAPIST: So, she tries to protect everybody—regulates the amount of pain that she thinks that each person in the family can tolerate at any given moment.

MOTHER AND FATHER (*respond in unison*):   Exactly!

MOTHER: I'll give you an example. My nephew was having a hard time. He had severe ADHD [attention-deficit/hyperactivity disorder], and I know that my sister and brother-in-law were going through a lot with him, a lot of worries.

THERAPIST: And did your sister ever turn to you to share, to get support?

MOTHER: No, we all keep our troubles to ourselves. I don't want to be intrusive.

THERAPIST: If she were to come to you and let you in, would you want to be there for her?

MOTHER: Sure. I know it would ease her distress. Help her feel less alone.

THERAPIST: It seems like in your efforts to protect one another, you all keep your emotions pretty private but that this leads to being alone and not being able to support each other.

MOTHER (*nods "yes" and begins to tear up*): I think she doesn't want to upset or burden me. Just like I don't want to burden her or my mother. I know that if I tell them about Alex, they will be upset. But I know that we need to find the way to break through this obstacle, this blockade.

THERAPIST: What do you mean by breaking through the "blockade"?

MOTHER: To expose ourselves. To stop avoiding. To have more open conversations in the family and start sharing with a wider circle of people. I want to reach that point where it doesn't feel like it is so difficult. The point where I feel more at peace with Alex being gay. I just need to find a way to feel comfortable enough to open up to others about it.

FATHER: I have reached the point where I don't care what friends or family say. I know that most of them will be accepting and, the other half . . . that is their problem.

THERAPIST: If somehow you could both be more open and share. Get support from those family members and friends who are likely to be accepting. Is that something you would like?

FATHER: Yes. I think we just need the guts to come out and say, "That is us, this is our family, it is normal, and that is just the way it is!"

THERAPIST: Who are the people in the family you think would be the most accepting? Who could you turn to first if you were ready?

FATHER: Eileen's younger brother, his wife, all of the cousins. They have had Alex and his partner over for dinner. For them, it is really no big deal.

THERAPIST (*turns to mother*): Do you feel the same way? That your brother would react positively?

MOTHER: I agree. I don't think that they have a problem with Alex being gay.

THERAPIST: Can the two of you imagine inviting them over or meeting somewhere and telling them that you have been wanting to talk openly about Alex for a while but just haven't been able to do it? That you didn't want to burden them or make them feel uncomfortable, or that you were embarrassed?

MOTHER: I think it will be hard. We just have to find the right time. But, yes. I know that I need to do that. Not only for myself but for Alex. He has been begging us to be open with everybody. He constantly tells us that if we just talk to people, we will realize how much of a nonissue it is.

Returning to the case example of Maya introduced in Chapter 4, this next example was taken from the first alliance building session with Maya's parents. Her father, John, attributes his difficulty disclosing his daughter's minority identity to his continued hope that she might, one day, choose to be in a relationship with a man. He also mentions being dissuaded by his friends' homophobic attitudes. On the other hand, Maya's mother, Debbie, describes wanting to be more open about her daughter's identity and about her own feelings. At the same time, she wants to respect and protect her husband:

FATHER: We haven't shared information about Maya's identity, or her having a girlfriend, because of me. I didn't want anybody to know. I had hoped that it was a passing phase and that she would, in the end, be with a man.

THERAPIST: And today, are you still secretive about it?

FATHER: Yes. I don't share it with anybody. Maya is also discreet about it. She doesn't put things on Facebook or on other social media. And I don't bring it up or push.

MOTHER: I talk with my friends about many personal things but not about Maya and her sexual orientation.

FATHER: We men, in general, don't talk about things like that. I have a set of friends that I meet with regularly in the gym. We talk about all kinds of things—our marriages, our children. But ever since Maya has been in a relationship with a woman, I don't join those conversations. I just sit and listen. They don't know that Maya is bisexual. One of the guys in our group has a son who is gay. I hear the jokes the other guys make about gay people, even when he is around. It is even worse when he isn't there. So, I don't see the point.

THERAPIST: So, you feel like putting yourself out there and telling them about Maya would just make you the butt of their jokes. That nothing positive would come of it. That they wouldn't be supportive.

FATHER: Yes. Why open yourself up? In my opinion, it is still premature. I think that it's not right to decide for Maya. I think she hasn't made a final decision about her identity. If somebody asks me directly, however, I am going to be honest. I will say that, right now, she is with a woman, and if she is with a man in the future, so be it . . .

MOTHER: The hardest part for me is keeping it secret, not telling my friends. I know that they would be supportive. There are already two children in our group of friends who have come out. It's not new. I am not worried about how people will react. Quite the opposite. I know that they will be supportive. I just don't talk about it because of him [her husband].

THERAPIST: And would it make things easier for you if you were able to just open up and be honest and not have to conceal this secret from your friends?

MOTHER: Yes. It doesn't feel good walking around keeping a secret from my close friends.

THERAPIST: It seems like the two of you are in two different places in terms of telling your friends and family about Maya—that for you, John, it feels threatening and that nothing good will come of it. But for you, Debbie, it would bring a sense of relief and an opportunity to get support. (*Speaks to John*) Did you know that Debbie felt this way? That it was hard for her to keep this secret? That she would prefer to share with her friends and get support?

FATHER: To be honest, I didn't know that it was such a big deal for her. (*Turns to his wife*) If it is that important for you, as far as I am concerned, you can tell whoever you like. I'd rather you wait before you tell Esther, at least until I tell Tal [their friends], but the others. . . . That is fine with me. If there are ricochets, I know how to deal with them. I am not afraid.

PARENTS' OWN ATTACHMENT HISTORY AND
INTERGENERATIONAL RELATIONAL PATTERNS

After exploring parents' support system and the degree to which each parent is able to reach out to ask for support, the therapist dedicates one or two sessions to hearing about each parent's attachment history. More specifically, we ask each parent to share their experience of growing up in their family of origin. In particular, we are interested in the degree to which parents felt safe enough to share their feelings and needs with their own parents and could go to them for support and comfort during times of distress.

In some cases, parents describe loving, caring, open relationships with their parents. They portray their parents as having been accepting and positively involved in their life and as having provided support and protection, when necessary. They report that their parents were attuned to their emotions and needs and that they felt safe and secure, free to be themselves. In other cases, however, parents describe growing up in homes in which their parents were defensive, unavailable, secretive, fragile, critical, controlling, or even abusive. These parents learned that expressing vulnerability, assertive anger, and unmet needs was unsafe and only left them feeling worse. They recount feeling sad, frustrated, scared, and alone.

The purpose of helping parents reflect on and connect to their own attachment history is to use their experience as an empathic bridge to help them better understand their young adult's experience. With those parents who report having had a good relationship with their own parents during childhood—feeling validated, admired, and protected and being able to use their parents for support—therapists ask if they think that their young adult feels the same way. We ask if they think that their young adult feels like they can come to them for support and validation, including when they are feeling frustrated, hurt, and rejected by their responses to their sexual orientation or gender identity. Among the families we see, the answer to this question is usually "no" or "not regarding their being gay or transgender." In such cases, the therapist offers the treatment as an opportunity for parents to provide their young adult with the type of experience that they had as children: feeling secure, connected, respected, and able to share their feelings and know that they will be heard and taken seriously.

With those parents who report having had a poor attachment relationship with their own parents, therapists offer treatment as an opportunity to give their young adult something different, something that they themselves had needed as children or young adults but did not get. We offer the treatment as an opportunity to help them help their young adult feel safe and sufficiently secure to express their authentic self, vulnerable emotions, and unmet needs and know that they will be met with empathic, supportive, validating responses, and a sense that everything is all right.

To begin this exploration, the therapist asks parents to think back to moments in their own childhood or young adulthood when they felt ashamed, scared, alone, or otherwise in distress. We ask them to connect to what they needed from their parents in those moments and how their parents responded. The goal in this phase is not to exhaustively gather details about every life event. Instead, the therapist is looking for paradigmatic examples that reflect the degree to which parents could or could not turn to their own parents, be vulnerable, and get the support, comfort, recognition, validation, and sense of safety they so needed.

In families with two parents (or caregivers), therapists do this work with both parents in the room. We first focus on one parent's family history and then on the other parent's family history. Our experience is that when working with one parent, the other parent is almost always attentive and supportive. Moreover, the more that a given parent shares painful memories, the more empathic the other parent becomes. Frequently, the witnessing parent will move closer to their partner, reach out to physically support them, or make comments that validate their partner's experience. Sometimes the witnessing parent hears things or understands things that they did not know or understand previously, and their compassion for their partner increases. Indeed, we have found that even with parents whose relationship is tense or conflictual, being in the room while their partner talks about their attachment history is not only possible but often promotes intimacy and caring.

The therapist typically starts the session by explicitly saying,

> Today, I want to take some time to hear a little bit about the families each of you grew up in. What it was like in your family, what your relationships with your parents were like, and how things got talked about.

Some parents give brief responses (e.g., "My family was just a regular family. We all got along fine"). In such cases, the therapist needs to prompt the parent to get a fuller, more detailed attachment narrative. Other parents offer extensive, highly reflective, and rich descriptions of their childhood experiences with their parents and how those experiences have affected their parenting and relationship with their young adult.

In the following excerpt, Alex's mother speaks about how she refrained from sharing things with her own mother to protect her, and how, in turn, this dynamic has been replicated in her relationship with Alex, who avoids sharing his feelings with her in an effort to protect her:

THERAPIST (*speaks to mother*): Eileen, when you were growing up and you had a hard time, when something happened in your personal life with friends, perhaps a romantic partner, or at school. Did you share those kinds of thing with your parents?

MOTHER: No, I never really told my parents about those kinds of things. My father was away a lot. He was in the military, and we sometimes didn't see him for weeks at a time. I didn't tell my mother about what was going on with me. She would just become upset, and it was more stressful for me than helpful. I didn't want to hurt or burden her.

THERAPIST: So, who did you tell? Who helped you through those difficult times?

MOTHER: Nobody, really. I learned to deal with things myself.

THERAPIST: That sounds hard, lonely.

MOTHER: Sometimes it was. But that is just the way it was.

THERAPIST: Were there times when you wished you had somebody to share things with, somebody you could go to so that you didn't feel all alone?

MOTHER: Yes. I had an aunt that I could talk to sometimes, but she lived far away, and we only saw each other from time to time. My mother just wasn't that kind of person.

THERAPIST: Your aunt—she was somebody who you could confide in? Somebody who you could talk to when things were tough or complicated?

MOTHER: Yes. She was kind of the mother I never had.

THERAPIST: I was wondering if you think that Alex, to some extent, also hesitates to come to you for support sometimes because he is afraid to cause you pain? That sometimes he chooses to protect you the way that you protected your mom instead of telling you when he is down or frustrated? That perhaps he keeps things to himself?

MOTHER: Definitely. I see that he is worried about me all of the time. He constantly asks me how I am doing. In some ways, he is exactly like me. Because he doesn't want to hurt us, he has distanced himself from us. With his friends, he has open, loving, close relationships. With us, he is careful . . . I know that it is hard for him because he knows that when he shares with me things related to his being gay, it hurts me (*begins to cry*), and that is hard for him.

THERAPIST: Because he loves you so much, he is afraid to hurt you?

MOTHER (*nods "yes"*): Yes. I know how much he cares about me and is afraid to hurt me. He has always been protective of me. He can't see me in a situation that is stressful for me or where I will be hurt. But I am strong enough to take care of myself. I don't need him to protect me.

THERAPIST (*turns to father*): David, what is it like hearing Eileen talk about these things?

FATHER: It's true. I have known Eileen's mother for 30 years. She is a wonderful, generous woman. She loves Eileen more than anything in the world. But she can't tolerate pain. If somebody is in distress, is suffering, she is the last person they will go to. I can see why Eileen has learned to deal with things alone, quietly.

THERAPIST: But this leaves her in distress.

FATHER: Absolutely. I try to support her the best I can.

THERAPIST: So, in those moments, does she come to you for support?

MOTHER: David wants to be there for me. It is really more about me withdrawing. I know that if I want support, he will be there in a minute.

THERAPIST: Okay. We will get back to this a little later. We can talk more about how the two of you can work together so that you, Eileen, don't end up in corner feeling alone. . . . Going back to Alex, I can hear how much he loves you and wants you to feel good. But I also imagine that he has paid, and is still paying, a big price for that. That, much like you did when you were younger, he keeps a lot inside and is afraid to come to you for support or even just share his feelings and needs. It also sounds like it has taken a toll on the relationship. That instead of being close and sharing with you, he has kept his distance.

MOTHER: I know that. I can see that he holds back and doesn't really tell what is going on in his life.

THERAPIST: Is that something that you would like him to know—that you are strong enough? That he doesn't need to protect you the way that you had to protect your mother, and that you do want to be there for him to hear what is going on in his life and support him the best you can?

MOTHER: Absolutely! I am his mother.

THERAPIST: Great. That is something I am going to help you do when we all meet together: let him know that you want to hear what is going on with him and let him know that you are strong enough.

This next example is from the Gold family with Adam, a 28-year-old gay man, in his last year of nursing school. His father, Moshe, worked in sales, and his mother, Ruth, was a court clerk. In the segment that follows, Moshe and Ruth talk about the messages that they received from their own parents: that one should hide their weaknesses, cover anything that might seem like a liability, and generally not talk about emotions:

FATHER: My mother always said, "Don't let anybody know that you have a learning disability." My parents never asked for help, never asked for medical or psychological services.

MOTHER: They were refugees from the war. They were self-reliant. It was against their values to ask for help. You take care of things by yourself, keep it to yourself.

THERAPIST (*speaks to father*):   And what about you? Were you open about your having a learning disability?

FATHER: I didn't tell anybody. I learned that you have to hide things. That's what I learned from my mother, from my father. I never went to ask for help or special treatment. I kept it to myself. Adam, our son, always tells me that that is where my attitude comes from. That I am used to hiding things about myself from others, and that is why I hide his homosexuality and expect him to do the same. He connects between those two things.

MOTHER: That is the mentality we grew up with. To sweep things under the rug. In my family, things were also kept from us. I grew up in a family in which I never saw my parents fight or tension between them. Then, one day, I get a call to come home immediately, and my father announced that he was leaving the family. I was in shock. I had no idea.

THERAPIST: This "sweeping things under the rug, hiding things" . . . it sounds hard?

MOTHER: Yes! For me, there was no preparation. No time to talk about feelings, to get used to things.

THERAPIST: Did you feel like it would have helped if things were out in the open, talked about.

MOTHER: Yes.

THERAPIST: I can see where you both learned to hide things, keep them to yourselves. Do you think that Adam also wished things were more out in the open? That he could talk to you more about his personal life? That the two of you would feel more comfortable letting people know that he was gay?

FATHER: Absolutely. He said that that is one of the things that most bothers him. That we hide the fact that he is gay. He says that it has made him self-conscious.

THERAPIST: Okay. That is one of the things we are going to talk about when we all get together for joint sessions.

PROCESSING PARENTS' EMOTIONS ABOUT HAVING A SEXUAL OR GENDER MINORITY CHILD

In the next phase of this task, therapists invite parents to talk about what it has been like for them trying to come to terms with having a sexual or gender minority child. The purpose of this exploration is to help parents access and work through their maladaptive emotions, including global distress, rejecting anger, internalized shame, and excessive fear that are fueling their nonacceptance. For many parents, this is the first time they have ever spoken to anybody about their experience of having a sexual or gender minority child, and such sessions can be highly arousing.

ABFT-SGM therapists often begin by asking parents to recall episodic memories of when their child first came out or when they first learned about their child's orientation or gender identity. Some parents describe shock and fear, feeling like their whole word collapsed. Other parents are less surprised but still feel a pit in their stomach when they actually hear their child say the words "Mom, Dad, I am gay" or "Mom, Dad, I am trans" out loud. After recounting episodic memories of their child's coming out, parents typically continue by sharing other emotion-laden events, such as the first time their child was in a same-sex relationship, being asked by their child to refer to them using their chosen name or set of pronouns, seeing their child's physical appearance begin to change, or coming out to family members.

Most parents who come for ABFT-SGM still feel helpless and hopeless and are unable to let go of their heteronormative dreams or expectations. Some describe feeling like they have lost the child and the life they had or expected. This may be particularly true for parents of transgender young adults. Gender is a core organizing principle that informs who we are as people and our roles and ways of acting in relationships. This is especially evident in family relationships. A mother–daughter relationship is usually quite different from a father–son relationship. Thus, when a person comes out as transgender, their parents often experience a profound sense of loss and confusion (Wahlig, 2015). Biological sex and gender are so integral to personal identity that a change in one or both of them causes family members to feel that the person has fundamentally changed (Norwood, 2012). For most people, understanding the disconnect between a person's biological sex and gender identity can be challenging. For some parents, it is mind boggling (Pearlman, 2006).

Some parents are still preoccupied by questions about whether their young adult's sexual orientation or gender identity is genetically determined or a choice. They may be angry at their young adult for not "making better decisions" or "trying harder" to be straight or cisgender. Some wonder whether they themselves are responsible for their young adult's being gay or transgender. Most feel some degree of shame because they perceive their young adult as defective, damaged, or somehow less than. They feel that, by extension, they themselves and their entire family are also flawed. They also fear how others will react, including friends, colleagues, neighbors, and their own parents, siblings, and extended family. They are afraid of being pitied, devalued, or shunned. Many parents are also terrified about what the future holds for their young adult and imagine their child living their life alone, miserable, vulnerable, and exploited.

Using the framework of emotion theory (Safran & Greenberg, 1991), primary maladaptive shame and excessive fear are understandable but maladaptive responses to pernicious, disparaging societal homo(trans)phobic messages and stereotypes to which parents have been exposed all of their life (Greenberg & Iwakabe, 2011). Global distress, helplessness, and rejecting anger, on the other hand, are considered secondary, defensive emotions. They are reactions to, and attempts at regulating, the painful primary maladaptive emotions of shame and fear. Both primary maladaptive and secondary emotions are unhelpful because they do not inform parents about what they need to feel better (e.g., to grieve their loss of the heteronormative dream, be reassured, get support, set limits with others, know that others still respect them). Moreover, their associated action tendencies (e.g., to shrink and withdraw, to hide) do not help parents get their needs met. It is quite the opposite. Hiding and withdrawing only reinforce and amplify parents' fear and shame, creating a vicious cycle. Likewise, parents' rejecting anger of their young adult's sexual orientation or gender expression leads the young adult to feel resentment. This, in turn, leads the young adult to either attack or disengage, which then leads to increased parental criticism and control. This negative cycle only deepens the relational rupture.

Pascual-Leone and Greenberg (2007) suggested that productive emotional processing is sequential in nature. It involves helping people move from highly aroused secondary emotions with low levels of meaning (i.e., global distress, rejecting anger) to more differentiated, personally meaningful but still maladaptive emotions, such as excessive fear and internalized shame. This then provides access to more adaptive emotions, such as adaptive grief and assertive anger. In the context of ABFT-SGM, grief is adaptive because it accurately signals to parents that they have experienced loss (e.g., the heteronormative future they expected and were invested in, the child they thought they had, their social status and self-worth). Adaptive grief also signals to parents that they need comfort and reassurance, which increases the likelihood that they will reach out for support from others.

Assertive anger is adaptive because it signals to parents that they have unfairly been made to feel broken, inadequate, and as if something wrong with them and their young adult. It elicits in them a healthy, legitimate demand from the environment that they and their young adult be treated as normal, equal, and with respect. Assertive anger also leads parents to set boundaries with others, including standing up to others when they make homophobic or transphobic comments, and advocate for their young adult's rights. When parents fully access their adaptive emotions, including pride and assertive anger, they feel a sense of relief and agency. They become more available and committed to hearing, validating and meeting their young adult's needs in later stages of the treatment.

To facilitate productive emotional processing, ABFT-SGM therapists begin by empathically listening to parents' despair and rejecting anger without judgment. This is not always easy. Sometimes parents say hurtful, disparaging things about their young adult or their young adult's identity. Indeed, when parents feel safe enough and are not afraid of being judged, they may share previously unspeakable thoughts, such as wishing their child was never born. It is essential that parents feel comfortable enough to be honest and candid about their thoughts and emotions, and say them aloud, no matter how taboo they might be. Disowned and repressed thoughts and feelings cannot be processed and transformed. In these moments, the therapist needs to maintain a state of unconditional, radical empathy and acceptance. By remaining empathic and nonreactive, the therapist validates parents' distress while at the same time modulating their panic and arousal through coregulation. We find it helpful to keep in mind that no parent wants to feel this way about their child and that their responses come from a place of terror, helplessness, and despair.

Once parents' secondary emotions are activated, the therapist attempts to help them access more differentiated primary maladaptive emotions. This helps parents gain a clearer understanding of what is driving their distress. For example, after hearing parents speak in general, global terms about how their life has been ruined, the therapist might say, "I can see how hard all of this is for you. What is the hardest part?" Parents will often respond by describing more differentiated maladaptive emotions, such as shame and excessive fear. For example, a father might respond by saying, "I can't bring myself to tell anybody at work that my son is gay. I am ashamed. I know what they will think of me" or "I am afraid of what his life is going to look like. What are they going to think when he interviews for a job? Nobody is going to hire him."

Finally, after parents' primary maladaptive emotions (e.g., internalized shame, excessive fear) are activated, the therapist helps them access and connect to more adaptive emotions, such as adaptive grief and assertive anger. One way we do this is by tracking, attending to, and highlighting the less dominant but adaptive emotions just below the surface of parents' narratives. For example, parents may talk about feeling ashamed by the thought of having their daughter bring her same-sex partner to the next family event. At some point, we shift the focus to parents' underlying sense of loss that things did not turn out the way they had always hoped they would, that they will never feel the excitement and joy of getting to see their daughter sitting next to her cisgender husband and their two kids at the dinner table. When parents are able to access, articulate, and productively process their adaptive grief associated with their loss, and let go of their heteronormative or gender-normative dream, their natural, adaptive instinct to create a new, positive vision of their future arises.

Likewise, when parents talk about their shame and fear about how their own parents, friends, or community may respond negatively to their child's minority identity, the therapist asks parents to describe exactly what they imagine that others will think, say, and do. When parents describe these anticipated negative responses in detail, one of two things typically happens. Either the parent themselves, or their spouse, recognize that their fears are excessive or unfounded, tempering their anxiety and concerns. Alternatively, saying out loud the biased, unjust, hurtful things parents imagine or fear that others will say and do elicits in parents' a sense of rightful indignation. Such indignation activates in parents a natural, adaptive instinct to stand up for themselves and their young adult, set clear limits with others, and demonstrate pride in their young adult.

In the following example, the therapist works with Alex's mother, Eileen, who is in a state of severe global distress. She came to the first alliance-building session feeling like her world had fallen apart. She felt helpless. She described how feelings of dread and hopelessness would suddenly and unexpectedly wash over her at various points during the day. In the following excerpt, the therapist works to help her disentangle and differentiate between the conglomeration of negative emotions fueling her high level of global distress. Alex's father, David, on the other hand, begins this same segment talking about his shame. Over the course of the conversation, he gradually accesses his feelings of loss and adaptive grief:

THERAPIST: Eileen, I want to try to help you put your finger on what specifically is hardest for you.

MOTHER: It is not any one single thing.

THERAPIST: I see that. So, let's talk about all of the different things, one at a time, to tease it all apart.

MOTHER: I don't know. Whenever I think of one thing in particular, I say to myself that it is not the end of the world. For example, when I imagine Alex coming home for Friday night dinner with a partner, I know that in the end, I will be fine. That everybody will accept it as being normal. I know that. But it is hard for me to reach that point in my mind.

THERAPIST: When you imagine that situation, what makes it so hard for you?

MOTHER: I guess what bothers me is that things are imperfect. That people will think that there is something wrong with our family. That there is something wrong with me. I know that nobody is perfect. But things were always in my control. In this case, I can't change him. Everything else in our lives, we decided. We decided and had the choice. We always aimed high. I always had the confidence that my kids would do well, would succeed.

And it always turned out the way I imagined. All of us have reached whatever goals we set for ourselves. In this case, there is something that is not normative in my family, and I have no control over it.

THERAPIST: So, the hard part is feeling like something is wrong with Alex? That his sexual orientation is a blemish, a failure, a mark on both him and the family?

MOTHER: I know that it is *us* who have to go through a process, to cope with our own homophobia. Consciously, I know what I need to do. Unconsciously, I feel like I can't let go. All of the things that I was afraid of months ago, that others will look down on him and on us, I know that they are not real. Every interaction I have with others proves that I don't really have anything to worry about in reality. Friends are accepting, family is accepting. I just have a hard time letting go.

FATHER: And what makes this so hard is that he is the most important thing in the world to us, a part of us. You know, when it is somebody else's child, it doesn't seem so tragic. But when it is your child . . . first, I started to wonder, "What did I do wrong?" Maybe I could have done something so that he wouldn't have turned out that way. Then I started to research on the internet: Where does it come from? What causes it? In the generation I grew up in, it is something terrible. I don't know what is worse, having a gay child or a seriously ill child. It is something where others look at us and say, "Look at that poor man. What a terrible tragedy befell his family."

THERAPIST: As if something is wrong with your son, and in turn, the whole family.

FATHER: Yes, like he is defective. I invested everything I have in him . . . (*begins to tear up*).

THERAPIST: What is happening inside of you right now?

FATHER: Disappointment. I feel like I lost what might have been, what should have been. Ever since he was a child, I have seen him as a copy of myself, but a better version of myself. I am looking for a way to be at peace with this defect and live with it. You know, Alex has so many great qualities. He is an amazing person. You should see how many friends he has who love him. He is one of the most appreciated people at his workplace.

THERAPIST: He sounds special, loved, successful. I hear that it is hard for you to let go of certain expectations and hopes, but I also hear that there is so much about Alex to be proud of.

In the next example, Natalie's father, who is religious, begins by talking about his maladaptive fears—his fear that his daughter's sexual orientation will reflect poorly on his own standing in the community and on the family and his fear that her minority identity will negatively affect her siblings, including her three sisters' ability to find an appropriate wedding match. Over the course of this segment, the therapist works to help the father access assertive anger. Also, at the end of the segment, both the mother, Sarah, and father, Jacob, begin to come in contact with their sense of loss and adaptive grief:

THERAPIST: I can hear how essential you feel it is to keep Natalie's identity secret, even in your own family, and your fear about what might happen if people in your community find out—that it may impact on how you are perceived.

FATHER: Absolutely. I think about that a lot. It is not like we live in a society where she will be shunned or people will stop talking with us, but it will definitely be juicy gossip.

THERAPIST: What do you think people will say?

FATHER: I have two thoughts. First, there will be those who will gloat. They will say, "He is not as good as he thinks he is. Life is not so perfect for him." Second, there will be those who will say, "This is what happens when you raise your children too liberally."

THERAPIST: That is upsetting, feeling like you are going to be judged negatively by others.

FATHER: And it is not just about me. If people realize that Natalie is a lesbian, it is going to make it harder for her sisters to find good matches. Any way you look at it, it is a blemish on the family.

THERAPIST: Wow. That is so unfair. It is also complicated. On the one hand, there is your desire to be good parents—support and accept your daughter and help her feel good about herself. On the other hand, you are afraid about the consequences of her coming out publicly on your personal life and the lives of your other children.

A little later in the same session:

THERAPIST (*speaks to mother*):   I saw that you began to tear up.

MOTHER: As I am listening to the conversation, one of things I think we have done over the past few years is practice denial. I think we have repressed our feelings of loss and grief. Now that we are here, it reminds me of how sad we felt in the past, in the beginning. We speak about it less now, but a year ago, we talked about it more explicitly. It was more present in our lives. I remember us saying things like, "People who have lost their child, everybody knows and comes and comforts them, and they sit shiva." With us, we also lost our child, but nobody knows. It's just between us. In some ways, it is mourning, but it is mourning something that didn't happen. Something inside of us is mourning, but in reality, we are not in mourning (*both parents pause and reflect*). Another thing that I think we repress, and this is even sadder, is . . . "Who is this girl that we lost?" On the one hand, you can say that we never really knew her. That she had all of this going on inside, and it was just a facade, not really her. On the other hand, from an early age, we were so connected. She was loving, articulate. We couldn't get enough of each other. We sat and talked and read.

FATHER: Yes. We used to talk all of the time. All of that disappeared. Natalie and I were always very close, a special and strong relationship. This loss is very hard for me, this distance and tension in the relationship. She was one of the few people in the world I felt like I could talk with, and we would understand each other perfectly. It was always a pleasure speaking with her.

THERAPIST: It sounds really special, this relationship each of you had with Natalie. That is really a big loss. I am sure that a large part of that relationship was real, even if she didn't share certain parts of herself. She is still the same person with all of those wonderful qualities.

FATHER: Yes (*begins to tear up*).

MOTHER: (*Also begins to cry*).

THERAPIST: That is a big loss.

PROMOTING PARENTAL REFLECTIVE FUNCTIONING

After helping parents productively process their global distress, rejecting anger, fear, and shame, and get more in touch with their adaptive grief and assertive anger, the therapist shifts the focus of the session once again. They invite parents to reflect on how their nonacceptance has affected their young adult and their relationship with their young adult. This shift is a critical step in ABFT-SGM. It redefines the problem for parents. Instead of focusing primarily on their own difficulty coping with their young adult's minority identity, this shift invites them to focus on how they have hurt, and are still hurting, their young adult and are pushing them away. It redirects parents' attention away from their own experience and onto their young adult's experience.

In many cases, parents already have some idea of how their nonaccepting behaviors and their own anger, shame, and excessive fears have caused their young adult pain. However, now that parents have partially worked through some of their maladaptive emotions, and their level of distress has decreased, they are more able and willing to reflect on their young adult's experience. They are in a softer, more regulated, less defensive, and more open state. They can consider their young adult's thoughts, feelings, needs, and desires. This is what Fonagy et al. (1991, 1998) termed *reflective functioning* or *mentalization*: parents' ability to envision their child's internal mental states and reflect on how their own internal mental experiences have shaped and changed their interactions with their child (Luyten et al., 2017).

When parents are able to effectively imagine their young adult's experience of hurt, loneliness, shame, loss, grief, fear, and anger caused by feeling unaccepted, and recognize what their young adult needed and still needs from them, parents become more empathic toward their young adult. Feelings of sadness and regret begin to surface. Parents begin to more fully connect to the pain and suffering that their young adult has endured, and their natural instinct to reach out to their young adult to better understand and meet their needs is activated. Parents become motivated to be there for their young adult in a more responsive manner (Strifler et al., 2022).

Once parents are more aware of, and in touch with, the toll that their nonacceptance has had on their young adult and the relationship, and they are motivated to be more accepting and responsive, the therapist explicitly offers relational repair as the primary goal of the therapy. Typically, the therapist says something like this:

> If I could help you reach out to your daughter in a way that would help her to open up, both about some of the things that have happened in the past and

about how she feels in the relationship now—so that the three of you could work through some of the past hurts and think about what she needs to feel more accepted and connected now—would that be a good goal for you?

Almost always, by this stage in the treatment, the answer to this question is an emphatic "Yes. That is why we are here."

In the following example, Maya's parents recount how they responded to their daughter when she first came out and over the ensuing years. They are able to reflect on how their negative responses must have caused their daughter pain. This recognition elicits in them adaptive shame and regret, which then motivate them to want to repair the relationship.

FATHER: I know that I hurt her terribly and that she is still carrying around feelings about what happened.

THERAPIST: Can you say more?

FATHER: I think that she is still carrying with her the shock that, in the blink of an eye, her father basically disconnected from her. Looked at her with disdain. Rejected her. The fact was that I was willing to disconnect from her if that was the way she was going to be. I was stupid. I thought that if I made her choose between being with a woman or having a relationship with me, then she would choose our relationship. I remember how she sobbed. I intentionally put her in the position that she had to choose one or the other in an effort to influence her.

MOTHER: When she was 14, she had a girlfriend. John told her that she had to end that relationship. That she couldn't bring her home anymore. She was very upset. There was lots of crying and drama around that event. In the beginning, John felt that if he blocked her from seeing her girlfriend, he could actually prevent Maya from becoming a lesbian. I was afraid we were going to lose her, and I found myself in the middle, trying to temper his responses.

FATHER: I think our nonacceptance led to her dysregulation, to her extreme moods, uncontrolled panic attacks. Look, we neglected her. We didn't see her distress. We weren't there for her. We gave her the cold shoulder. I gave her the cold shoulder. Today, we know that she was in real distress. We didn't accept her girlfriends. It was a bad period. A lot of bad blood flowed then. We got caught in a negative cycle.

MOTHER:	Then, for 3 years, she was with a boyfriend, and we thought, "It is over. It is in the past." We forgot all about it. But at one point, that relationship just ended. Then, not so long afterward, Maya told me, "You know, the whole thing with women may be relevant again in the future." At one point, she was in a relationship with another woman, and we found out through indirect means. From that time on, it felt like she was uncomfortable, embarrassed . . . and then there was a parade of one boy after another. Each one for a week, 2 weeks, and then these relationships would end. Again, we thought her feelings for girls had passed, and then she met Ariel. She brought her to dinner once, and it was very hard for us to talk to her. Maya accused us of acting differently when she was with a woman than when she was with a man. I told her, "Yes, you are right."
THERAPIST:	So, she felt like it was hard for you, uncomfortable, when she was in a relationship with a woman.
MOTHER:	I felt like the whole situation was artificial.
FATHER:	I am not going to lie. When I see two women together, I feel disgusted, repulsed.
MOTHER:	I also feel that way. When we went to a wedding with two men, it was hard for me to watch.
THERAPIST:	And Maya picks up on that? It affects her?
FATHER:	Maya and Ariel make sure not to have any physical contact when I am around. I remember one time, they had come over to the house, and I walked into the living room, and Maya had her arm around Ariel. I almost lost it. I have to work on myself. It is really, really hard for me not to react. I am jealous of people who can tolerate and accept, but it is hard for me.
MOTHER:	I think that the feeling of being a disappointment to her father weighs very heavy on her . . . she feels like she failed him. It is internalized deep inside of her?
THERAPIST (*turns to father*):	Do you also think that Maya is afraid that you are disappointed in her?
FATHER:	She wants me to be proud of her. And she knows my attitude, and I think she takes that into consideration.

MOTHER: I also think she was disappointed that I didn't support her more during that time. That I didn't confront John and take her side. Also, I was so cold and detached when she brought her girlfriend home. I told her that I am willing to accept her relationship with her girlfriend, but that I am not happy like I would be with a man. I was honest with her.

FATHER: We let Maya down in a big way!

MOTHER: I think because she sees it is hard for us to come out to others, she is more careful, more hesitant to be herself. Deep down, I think she is afraid of being hurt by our reactions, disappointed by us again.

THERAPIST: And how do you think that affects her inside?

MOTHER: I know it causes her anxiety, stress. She wants us to be proud of her, just like any child wants their parents to be proud of them. She is constantly worried that we will flip out or that we pull away from her again.

THERAPIST: That at any point she might lose her relationship with one or both of you? That she can't be sure that you will be there for her, support her, continue to appreciate her, regardless of who she is with?

MOTHER: Yes. And that is not fair to her. It is not fair that she has to walk around feeling like that. Feeling like something is wrong with her.

FATHER: I want her to know that I am in a different spot today. It may be hard for me. But I want her to be happy. To make her own choices. I don't want her to feel like she needs to hide anything from us anymore.

THERAPIST: Have you guys ever talked with Maya about how she felt during those times in the past, when she was afraid or alone, or how she feels today, seeing the disappointment in your eyes?

FATHER: Not really.

THERAPIST: Do you think she is still carrying around some of those bad feelings or still harbors fears that, like in the past, you might reach a point where you become angry again and cut off from her?

FATHER: I don't know, but if she does, I want to turn over a new leaf. I want her to know that I am in a different spot today. It may be hard for me, but I want her to be happy. To make her own choices. I don't want her to feel like she needs to hide anything from us anymore.

THERAPIST: Okay. That is something I want to help you with. To invite Maya to share some of what it has been like for her since coming out, get it off of her chest, help you guys to work through those past memories. You know, sometimes we have to work through old hurts before we can begin to trust again, before we can move forward. I also want to help you guys check with her about how safe she feels today. What she needs from you to be open and share more. What she needs in order to feel closer and more connected to you both.

In the next example, Alex's mother responds to the therapist's question about whether she thought her global distress affected her son. She indicated that she thought her own difficulty accepting his sexual orientation led him to pull away from her, come home less frequently, and created distance in their relationship:

MOTHER: I know that my distress, fears, and secrecy make it harder for him. It forces him to lie, and that makes it hard on him. He needs to live his own authentic life, and we don't let him. It also probably impacts other aspects of his life, like work. It is hard for him to deal with his double life. He doesn't feel whole, neither in his day-to-day life nor at home. There are always secrets, situations in which he needs to check himself. Also, between us, we don't talk freely about everything. There is this constant stress, this monitoring of what is and what isn't said. We don't ask questions about the people in the pictures he puts up on Facebook. We avoid talking about lots of things. He also stops himself from talking about things. There are boundaries.

THERAPIST: Boundaries around what things?

MOTHER: Boundaries around everything because we are not sufficiently accepting. I can compare it to my daughter. Everything with her is much more open—about boyfriends, friends, her work— things are more open.

THERAPIST: And how do you think that it impacts Alex inside . . . your avoidance? That he sees you talking more openly with your daughter, asking more questions?

MOTHER: It impacts him a lot. I know that he very much wants to make us proud. And the fact that we don't ask him about his personal life, it makes him feel worse about himself. I know that he would want to be more open with us.

THERAPIST (*speaks to both parents*): So you think that he would want to be able to be more open with the two of you? To be able to share more about his personal life with you two?

FATHER: Yes, somewhat. At least a little bit more.

THERAPIST: And is that something the two of you would like? For Alex to be more open? To really know what is going on with him?

FATHER: Look, the whole point of these meetings is to be able to reach that state so that we can give him the feeling that we are there for him, with him. I am not going to say that it is easy.

THERAPIST: Okay. That is what I want to help you two do. I want to help you guys feel increasingly more comfortable—able to talk about and hear things that were too scary before. To give Alex the message that he can be more open. That despite it being hard for you, that you want to hear about and be more involved with his life. I think you are right. He wants you to know him and be proud of him.

PREPARING FOR SUBSEQUENT CONJOINT ATTACHMENT SESSIONS

Once parents are signed on to the goal of hearing more from their young adult about what it has been like for them over the years, and what they need now to feel accepted, supported, loved, admired, connected, and safe, the therapist prepares parents for the upcoming attachment task. Such preparation includes helping parents plan how to reach out to their young adult during upcoming conjoint sessions and how to listen. Preparing parents for these upcoming attachment sessions is essential for a number of reasons. First, it ensures that the content will be meaningful and will focus on the core relational themes and emotions fueling the young adult's experience of nonacceptance. By this point in the therapy, parents already have some understanding about what is upsetting their young adult. This includes past traumatic events and ongoing negative family dynamics. Parents also have some sense of what needs to change.

The therapist helps parents to explicitly articulate two or three events or themes that they know or imagine are bothering their young adult. They are asked to keep these events or themes in mind during upcoming attachment sessions as they reach out to their young adult. Although it is the young adult who will lead conversation when the family gets back together for conjoint sessions and will bring the material closest to their heart, this list of events and themes parents have prepared for themselves serves as a touchstone. It helps parents know when they and their young adult are talking about important things and the conversation is productive. It prevents the conversation from drifting off to tangential, banal, unrelated, or trivial content, and it serves as a road map for getting the conversation back on track, when necessary.

The second reason to prepare parents is because such conversations are often emotionally intense—laden with powerful affect. This may be the first time that parents witness the full extent of their young adult's vulnerability and pain or are the object of their young adult's adaptive anger for a sustained, uninterrupted period. This is challenging for most parents. In such moments, parents themselves may feel intense pain at seeing their young adult's pain. They also may feel guilty for not having done a better job seeing, supporting, or protecting their young adult. Some parents may also feel attacked.

For parents to be able to regulate themselves and respond optimally during such conversations, they need to be prepared ahead of time. The therapist does this by helping them imagine the upcoming conversations. The therapist asks parents to imagine what their young adult might say, how it will make them feel, and how they would like to respond. By imagining the conversation, parents are able to prepare their responses in advance—offline, when they are only moderately aroused. Such prepared responses are then ready to be retrieved and used in the heat of the moment. This reduces the risk that parents will become defensive, overwhelmed, or shut down during conjoint sessions.

In the following example, the therapist prepares a religious mother by inviting her to imagine how she would feel if her 21-year-old son were to tell her during the session that he has a boyfriend and does not want to have to hide that from her any longer:

MOTHER: I don't know how I would react. I know that it is going to come one day, but I don't know if I can handle it right now. In some ways, I would rather that he not tell me. I know that is unfair. I feel terrible about that. But, on the other hand, I don't know how I will react and if I will be able to cope.

THERAPIST: What are you afraid might happen in that moment?

MOTHER: I think my heart will sink. Just an empty feeling in my stomach. I will feel like all is lost, that it is final.

THERAPIST: It is good that we are talking about that now. That you can imagine the sense of loss and finality you might feel in that moment. . . . You also said earlier that despite all of your pain and fears, you want him to be able to come to you, to be open with you. If you could plan in advance how you would want to respond in that moment, what would that look like? How could you respond in a way that would make him feel that everything will be okay, that you are strong enough to handle this and want him to be open with you?

MOTHER: I would like to be able to tell him that I am happy for him. I don't want him to keep something like that from me and have no one to share it with. But, also, I can't pretend that I am not sad and worried.

THERAPIST: I think that is fine. I am not in favor of pretending. I think it is okay to say both of those things: that you are relieved or even happy that he has someone. That you don't want him to be alone. And, at the same time, that it is still hard for you. That you are still grieving the future you had imagined and that you are worried about his welfare. All of those things can be true at the same time.

Parents are often willing to face their fear and pain for the sake of their young adult and the relationship. Parents will do things for the benefit of their young adult that they would not have done otherwise.

It is also important to prepare parents so that the moment-by-moment process during attachment sessions goes well. Families are typically not used to, or skilled in, having deep, emotion-focused conversations about difficult, anxiety-producing topics. Therefore, therapists provide parents with some guidelines for approaching these sessions. This phase has a bit of a psycho-educational quality to it. We teach parents to act as *emotion coaches* (Gottman et al., 1996) who help their young adult to open up, access, and express their emotions and unmet needs. For example, we encourage parents to ask their young adult open-ended, experiential, and emotion-focused questions, such as, "How did you feel when we said that we didn't think we would be comfortable coming to your wedding?" We also encourage parents to ask their young adult what response they had hoped for or needed from them in a given moment or situation in the past. At the same time, we coach parents to refrain from behaviors that we know will interrupt their young adult's sharing and emotional processing. More specifically, we encourage parents to refrain from explaining things to their young adult, cross-examining them, lecturing, and arguing with them. Therapists present treatment as a unique opportunity for parents to put themselves aside momentarily and really hear and understand—perhaps for the first time—how their young adult feels and what they need.

Some parents are concerned that they will not have an opportunity to share their side of the story. They are concerned that the conversation will focus too much on their young adult's perspective, feelings, and needs and will not consider their own needs and the larger context. They fear that listening to and validating their young adult's experience and unmet needs implies that they agree with them and they are therefore obligated to meet all of their young adult's needs and demands.

To address parents' concerns, the therapist frames the upcoming attachment task as a two-step process. The first step involves fully hearing, understanding, empathizing with, and validating their young adult's experience of feeling rejected and what they need to feel more accepted and connected. The therapist first wants the young adult to feel heard, understood, validated, and supported. Then parents will have the opportunity to ask their young adult questions about things that, up until this point, seemed confusing to them. For example, they might ask their child why they did not tell them about their sexual orientation or gender identity earlier. Parents might also want to know why it is so important for the young adult to come out to their grandparents.

The therapist assures parents that in the latter part of the attachment task, they will have time to share their own experience of the relationship. When that time comes, parents may share how torn they feel wanting to support their young adult's identity while at the same time fearing that they will be ostracized by their own family. They may talk about their attempts to navigate between meeting their young adult's needs and other demands in their own lives. Some parents might want to talk about how hurt they feel when their young adult lashes out at them for no apparent reason and make it clear that they expect their young adult speak to them respectfully, even if they are frustrated. When parents are assured that, later in the task, they will have the opportunity to ask questions, talk about their own experience, and communicate their legitimate expectations from their young adult, they are more likely to be able to momentarily put themselves aside and be singularly focused on being there for their young adult.

In the last part of this preparation phase, the therapist assures parents that they will be there to support and guide them during upcoming conjoint attachment sessions to the degree necessary. The therapist also assures parents that, if need be, they will help them start the conversation with their young adult and redirect them if the conversation gets stuck or starts to escalate. The therapist explicitly asks for parents' permission in advance to intervene, when necessary. For example, the therapist will typically say something like the following:

> I am going to be there and will help if you need me. I also want to make sure that it is okay with you if I stop you, interrupt you, even in midsentence, if I see that things are escalating or going in the wrong direction. If I see that you are starting to get upset or are getting drawn into arguing with your daughter instead of trying to understand what she is trying to say.

When parents are on board with the goal of the attachment task, they welcome the therapist's offer of help. They themselves know that they may need help to regulate themselves, refrain from habitual negative responses, and stay on track. Getting parents' advanced permission to stop and challenge them in the service of facilitating new, more productive interactions is important in order to avoid potential ruptures in the therapeutic alliance and to maintain a shared, collaborative, goal-oriented focus.

6 THE ATTACHMENT TASK

The fourth task, the attachment task, is considered the pinnacle of the treatment. The purpose of this task is to facilitate corrective attachment episodes—the purported primary change mechanism of the treatment. During these in-session therapeutic enactments, the young adult and their parents have conversations about difficult topics in new and productive ways. This is in contrast to the past, when such conversations were either avoided or ended up leading to conflict and disengagement.

These new therapeutic conversations serve to help family members productively process past traumatic events and lingering negative feelings related to parents' rejection or nonacceptance of their young adult's identity. Corrective attachment episodes also serve to transform current negative interactional patterns fueling the young adult's sense of rejection.

Corrective attachment episodes begin with the young adult sharing with their parents, sometimes for the first time, their emotions (e.g., hurt, shame, fear, anger) associated with not feeling accepted as well as their unmet but legitimate attachment and identity needs (e.g., the need to be cared for;

https://doi.org/10.1037/0000352-006
Attachment-Based Family Therapy for Sexual and Gender Minority Young Adults and Their Nonaccepting Parents, by G. M. Diamond and R. Boruchovitz-Zamir

the need to be respected and validated; the need to feel worthwhile, a sense of belonging, and connected). The therapist then helps parents respond in an open, curious, empathic, validating, and caring manner. When parents respond in an attuned manner, the young adult feels heard, understood, validated, cared for, and safe. As a result, the young adult allows themselves to be increasingly vulnerable, further connecting to and elaborating on their emotions and unmet needs. This positive, cyclical process transforms the way that parents and their young adult relate and how they view and experience each other. When these conversations are successful, the young adult begins to see their parents as more available, understanding, and caring. At the same time, parents gain a better understanding of their young adult, what they have been through, and how their nonacceptance has negatively affected them. This process typically elicits in parents a sense of remorse and motivates them to want to better meet their young adult's needs. Tension in the relationship decreases; unresolved anger and hurt dissipate; positive feelings of love and closeness emerge; family members feel greater agency; and there is an increased sense of hope, trust, and security in the attachment relationship.

In attachment-based family therapy for sexual and gender minority young adults and their nonaccepting parents (ABFT-SGM), family members come to this task well prepared. The therapist has already spent time alone with the young adult during individual alliance building sessions, helping them identify some of the traumatic events, family dynamics and core relational themes fueling their experience of rejection. The therapist has also already helped them to begin connecting to and articulating their primary adaptive, but previously unexpressed, hurt and assertive anger associated with these traumatic events, negative dynamics, and feelings of rejection.

Likewise, the therapist has already met with parents alone during a series of alliance-building sessions. They have helped parents to process some of their shame and fear associated with having a sexual or gender minority young adult and reflect on their young adult's experience of their rejecting behavior. As a result, parents come to the session less distressed and more motivated to put their needs momentarily aside to hear and validate their young adult's experience and unmet needs. They also understand and are committed to the task at hand: to reach out to their young adult from a curious, open, empathic posture and avoid habitual defensive responses like lecturing, justifying their own behavior, or arguing with their young adult about the facts. This preparation, completed in previous tasks, increases the likelihood that the attachment task will be successful.

BEGINNING THE ATTACHMENT TASK

The attachment task begins with the therapist's ceremoniously marking the magnitude of the moment and the goal at hand (see Figure 6.1). After checking in briefly with family members about how they are doing, the therapist says something like this:

> Okay. This is a big day. I have spent a number of weeks meeting with each of you alone to help you prepare for this conversation. I am confident that you are ready. Today is an opportunity to talk about some of the topics that have been getting in the way of your relationship but have been hard to talk about up until this point.

ABFT-SGM therapists are aware that despite all the preparation, family members may be anxious. Parents may be worried that their young adult will get frustrated and lash out at them or shut down. They may also fear hearing painful or scary things that might lead them to feel pain, guilt, or concern for their young adult's well-being. The young adult, on the other hand, may be worried that the conversation will devolve into fighting like so many previous conversations. They may also be afraid that their parents will emotionally collapse, focus on their own feelings, or present themselves as victims. They fear, too, that their parents will blame them for being dramatic or selfish, invalidate what they say, or minimize their feelings, or that their parents will otherwise defend themselves. They are afraid that the conversation will be just more of the same—another in a long line of failed efforts to be heard, understood, appreciated, and accepted.

FIGURE 6.1. Structure of the Attachment Task

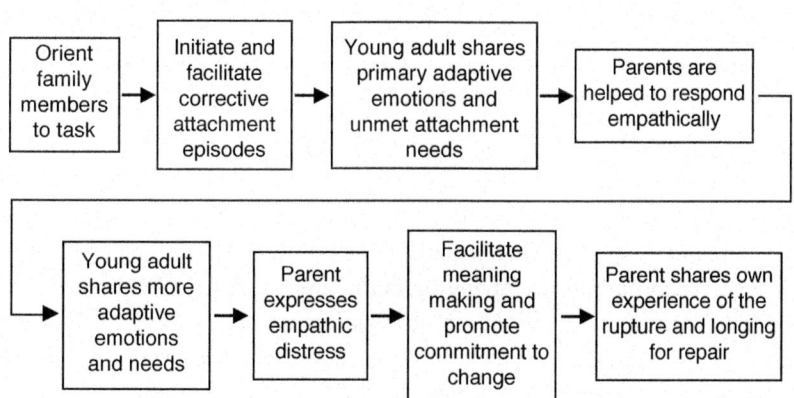

For all these reasons, the therapist promises that this conversation will be different, unlike interactions family members have had in the past. They create positive expectancy, instill a sense of confidence, and assure family members that they will be there to help them if they get stuck or go off track. The therapist says something like the following:

> I am here if you need me. If I feel like one of you needs some help, I will be there for you. Also, if I feel like you guys are getting stuck in some of the same old patterns, I will stop you, jump in, and help you get back to the things we marked as important in our sessions alone.

The therapist is confident that even if family members are unable to interact in an optimal manner during these first attachment sessions, they will be able to help them regulate themselves better, slow down, speak from a place of vulnerability and need, and avoid hurting or disappointing one another to the degree that they have in the past.

The therapist is less directive during the attachment task than during earlier tasks. Here, the process optimally occurs between family members. The goal is that the young adult and their parents engage in sustained, productive conversations about previously avoided and difficult topics, with the therapist intervening only when necessary. The therapist typically begins the task by inviting the young adult to start the conversation. Sometimes, a simple "Why don't you begin, Ron?" is enough. Other times, the young adult will initially look lost or ask for help to get started. At this point, the therapist might say, "Ron, maybe you could begin with one of the things we talked about during our sessions alone?" If the young adult needs further help, the therapist can be even more specific and concrete. For example, the therapist might say,

> When we met alone, Ron, you mentioned two things that really bothered you. One was the fact that you feel like your parents don't ask you about your personal life. The other was that you don't feel comfortable bringing Ido, your partner, to their house. Do you want to choose one of those topics?

If the young adult is really having a hard time, the therapist has the option of turning to their parents and asking them to invite their young adult to begin. This can be a powerful moment. When parents look at their young adult and ask them to share, it signals to the young adult that something has changed. Their parents are giving them the green light to talk about things that have been hard to talk about or off limits up until this point. Usually, this is enough to get the young adult started. Another way to get the conversation started is to have the parent introduce a topic they think their young adult might want to discuss. The therapist might say something like,

Dad, there were some things we talked about in our sessions alone that you thought might be bothering your son. Do you want to check in with him to see if one of those topics resonates with Ron and if he is willing to share his thoughts and feelings about it?

CONDUCTING CORRECTIVE ATTACHMENT EPISODES

Once the young adult begins to share, the therapist takes a step back and allows the conversation among family members to unfold. When the process goes well, family members turn toward and talk directly to one another rather than to or through the therapist. Parents carefully track their young adult. Ideally, they are attentive, nondefensive, and concerned. They ask their young adult for examples of specific events or interactions that best illustrate what is bothering them, and how they felt in those instances. Parents ask from a place of curiosity rather than to challenge or disconfirm their young adult's experience.

As their young adult shares, parents empathically validate their emotions. Again, this type of interaction is qualitatively different from past interactions. The young adult quickly notices that something essential has changed by the way their parents respond. Consequently, the young adult feels increasingly heard and safe and motivated to share more. When such conversations progress well, the therapist is an observer, a witness. Their job is to carefully monitor and contain the conversation. They intervene only when the family gets stuck; when the content becomes less meaningful; when the affect is off; or if one of the family members becomes overwhelmed, frustrated, or defensive and needs support, encouragement, or redirection. Ideally, the therapist does not need to intervene much. In practice, therapists may be required to be more active in the first session of this task and then incrementally less active as family members learn these skills and gain more confidence in having these types of conversations.

Returning to the case example of the Cohen family introduced in Chapter 3, the following examples are drawn from the first three attachment sessions with Natalie and her parents. In the first attachment session, the therapist introduces the attachment task, soothes Natalie's initial fears about the process itself, and then invites her to share with her parents her experience around the time she came out to them 2 years earlier:

THERAPIST: Okay. We have reached this moment which we have been working toward over the past few weeks. This is an opportunity
for the three of you to talk about some of the things that have

been hard to talk about before, that have come between you. I have met with each of you alone for a number of sessions, and you all have a good idea of some of the important things that you want to talk about. We will take it step by step. I'll be here to help if you get stuck, if you need support, and to keep things on track. Natalie, I know that you have a couple of things you wanted to bring up. Would you like to start?

NATALIE: I don't know exactly how to start (*long pause ensues*).

THERAPIST: We talked about a couple of things you might want to bring up. One was what went on, and how you felt, around the time you came out to your parents.

NATALIE: I am afraid.

THERAPIST: About what?

NATALIE (*pauses*):   To go back to that time . . . because it was very hard (*begins to tear up*). It is like going back into that same situation. And it is delicate and sensitive. The last time I tried it, 2 years ago, it ended badly.

Both of Natalie's parents look at her with concern and compassion. The therapist watches as Natalie registers her parents' empathic, supportive response:

THERAPIST: I appreciate your being so open about being scared. (*Turns to parents*) Mom, Dad. I wonder what is going through your minds and hearts when you look at Natalie right now and hear her fears?

MOTHER (*speaks directly to Natalie*):   Honey, that is why we are here. To talk about the things we haven't been able to talk about until now.

FATHER (*speaks directly to Natalie*):   Absolutely.

After getting her parents' permission, Natalie seems more ready. The therapist again turns to her to invite her to give it a try:

THERAPIST: The goal for today is to help you have a different experience. This time, we will try it together. I can see that your parents are here to listen. We will go slow. If it gets too difficult, we will take a pause and figure it out.

NATALIE (*alternates her gaze between her parents and the therapist*):   Okay. I think I'll start with the first time I told them. It was when I was away at college. I called on the phone. I called Mom and told her that there was something I wanted to tell her. I told her that I think that I am a lesbian. Meanwhile, the next thing I know, we are sitting in a therapist's office. The central message I heard coming from Mom and Dad was, "You are not a lesbian. You are not. You might think you are, but we know that you are not. You are just confused." (*With tears in her eyes, turns to her parents*) You gave a million reasons. You had this whole theory about why I am confused, and why I am mistaken, and why you think that I am not. That was the first message.

At this point, the therapist looks over at Natalie's parents to gauge their response. They seem attentive but tense. In light of Natalie's clear need to continue, the therapist decides not to intervene in this moment. Instead, the therapist monitors Natalie's parents' ability to continue to hear and contain Natalie's adaptive, assertive anger without resorting to defending themselves. Natalie continues talking:

NATALIE: And the second thing you said was, "Right now, the most important thing is that nobody finds out about this." That is what scared me most. And from that moment on, for a whole year, we didn't talk about it. And what I was left with, based on how you reacted, was that you don't believe it is true, and I must keep it a secret. And from that moment on, I felt like, okay, you don't really want to know who I am . . . because I come and tell you, and you don't listen. From that moment on, I thought, okay, why should I come and tell you anything?

As soon as Natalie pauses, the therapist turns to her parents to check in with how they are feeling, what is going on inside of them. Again, hearing their young adult's pain and grievances can be extremely hard and challenging for parents. It requires that they regulate themselves and keep their eye on the goal—understanding their young adult's experience. The therapist then speaks to Natalie:

THERAPIST: Okay. Let me stop you here for a second and check in with Mom and Dad. (*Turns to the parents*) Mom, Dad, did you know that was how Natalie experienced that whole event? Did you all ever talk about this?

FATHER: I didn't see it that way. That is not how I remember it happening.

DEALING WITH RESISTANCE

This is a critical point in the session. In this case, the young adult has just taken a chance and made herself vulnerable, expressing a mix of anger, fear, and helplessness. Her father, instead of maintaining an empathic, curious stance, becomes defensive and responds in a less than optimal manner. In this moment of empathic failure, the therapist must immediately step in to block and reshape the interaction. These early moments are when family members dare to test the waters of their relationship. They want to know whether the water is too hot or too cold, whether the undercurrents feel dangerous, or it is safe to go in deeper. Most importantly, they want to know whether there is a lifeguard on duty. That is why it is essential that the therapist quickly, sensitively, but assertively shape the process from the outset. If, in these first few minutes, family members feel unsafe or get hurt, they will leave the session feeling frustrated and hopeless about the therapy.

In the segment that follows, the therapist soothes the father's concerns about not having his side of the story heard, being vilified, or being unfairly judged. The therapist then redirects him back to the task at hand, which is trying to understand his daughter's experience and what she went through:

THERAPIST (*speaks to father*):　Jacob, I understand that your experience of what happened was different from that of Natalie's. We talked about this before when we met alone. Later in the sessions, it will be important to hear what it was like for you and what you remember. But right now, this is a unique opportunity for you to hear Natalie talk about what it was like for her—what she was thinking and feeling; what she is carrying around inside and what, for her, is getting in the way of the relationship today (*father nods in acknowledgment*). Can you ask her more about how that period felt for her?

FATHER:　I understand. I know that she felt disappointed in us, hurt by us. That we weren't open and didn't understand.

Again, the father does not ask Natalie about her experience. Perhaps asking questions is not his usual parenting style. Perhaps he is afraid of losing control. But productive enactments require that family members turn toward, and open up to, each other. This is how new information passes between them and new experiences are formed. Therapists want the parent to look into their young adult's eyes and say, "Tell me what it was like for you. I want to know how you felt." In the following segment, the therapist persists and asks the father to try again:

THERAPIST (*speaks to father*):   I know that you have some sense of what you think Natalie felt. This is a chance, however, for you to hear directly from her what it was like for her. Can you turn to her and ask her to say more about how she felt at the time so she knows that you really get it?

FATHER (*takes the therapist's direction and turns to Natalie*):   What was it like for you?

NATALIE: It destroyed me. Really. You guys didn't give me any place for me to be me. From that moment on, I felt like you didn't see me, you didn't know who I am. Like I have nothing. I have no home, no parents. It felt like . . . I am on one side, and you are on the other side. That I have to battle just so I can exist so that you don't erase me.

These moments, when a parent looks into their young adult's eyes and finally listens, hears, and understands the depth of their young adult's experience, can be powerful, affirming, and transformative for the young adult. Their experience of being heard is visceral. It is not just the words that their parents use to indicate that they hear and understand but also their facial expression, their gaze, their whole being.

As good as this moment is, the therapist must monitor that parents do not feel beaten up on. The young adult has a legitimate right to be disappointed and angry about being silenced, invalidated, or abandoned. However, there is a limit to how much sustained rejecting anger and blame parents can take, particularly this early in the process. Therefore, in these moments, the therapist needs to help the young adult access and express additional aspects of their emotional experience. This can be primary maladaptive emotions, such as fear and shame, or primary adaptive emotions, such as hurt and assertive anger, associated with feeling rejected. Some of this emotional processing work began earlier during individual alliance building sessions alone with the young adult. However, now, in the room with their parents, these emotions are even more accessible, salient, and intense:

THERAPIST (*speaks to Natalie*):   Can you tell them what else you felt?

NATALIE: Very alone. Scared.

MOTHER: And were you disappointed by our response in the sense that you had some expectation that we would react in a certain way, and we didn't?

NATALIE: I didn't think that it would be easy for you. I knew it wouldn't be simple for you. But you sat in front of me in the therapist's office and said, "I am not even able to say that word [lesbian], and I am not willing for you to say that word about yourself, either." That is a sentence that you said. I remember you said that, and my therapist remembers that you said it. The whole session, you weren't even willing to say the word "lesbian."

MOTHER: I just want to clarify that during that meeting, you didn't say you were a lesbian. You said you thought you might be a lesbian, and so . . .

NATALIE (*gets frustrated and raises her voice*): It doesn't matter exactly how I said it! That is not the point! I don't want to hear that or talk about that. I don't have to hear right now what was going through your minds. I want you to hear how very hard that period was for me. For once, please, put aside how hard it was for you, and listen to me. Try to understand what I was going through (*starts to cry*).

MOTHER (*catches herself and gets back to the task*): So, what was it like for you during that conversation?

NATALIE (*cries*): I don't want to tell you, anymore.

As this short segment shows, Natalie is beginning to access and express her fear and hurt. However, her mother responds in an unattuned manner. Instead of focusing on Natalie's fear and hurt and asking to hear more, she becomes defensive. She challenges the reasonableness of her daughter's expectations and disputes exactly what was or was not said. Understandably, this process is hard for the mother. Nevertheless, Natalie experiences her mother's response as an empathic failure. Consequently, she becomes frustrated and, in an effort to protect herself, shuts down. This brief interaction demonstrates how fragile this process can be in the beginning. The start of attachment episodes can be bumpy. Two steps forward, one step back. It is a process of successive approximation.

As the session continues, the therapist shifts the focus of the conversation to talk explicitly about the process itself and reflects the negative interactional cycle in which family members get caught:

THERAPIST: Natalie, I see how frustrated you are. I saw what just happened. You started to open up, and then Mom was more worried about clarifying what was or wasn't said than really listening and trying to understand how you felt in those moments. And then you got frustrated and shut down. And then, when Mom tried to correct herself, you had already checked out. (*Natalie nods "yes."*)

THERAPIST (*speaks to mother*): Did you see that cycle? (*Mother nods "yes."*) Okay. That's exactly what I want to help you all with: noticing when your responses kind of miss the mark and how to get back on track.

IDENTIFYING THE CYCLE

Helping family members see the negative interactional cycles that they get caught up in is a powerful intervention. Suddenly, they understand what is happening, and why. What once seemed like a mystery and inevitable now seems comprehensible and volitional. At this point, the therapist conveys to the family members that they have the power to change these cycles, to choose to respond differently:

THERAPIST (*turns to Natalie*): Like we talked about in our sessions alone, this process isn't easy. You guys have been stuck in this pattern for years. This therapy is an opportunity for you to transform your relationship. But it will not be easy. It is one step at a time. I want to challenge you a bit here, Natalie. Instead of throwing in the towel, I want you to try to give Mom another chance and see if she is able to listen now. (*Turns to mother*) Mom, this is your chance to try it again—to be singularly focused on Natalie's experience and to put aside for a moment how you remembered it or your urge to defend yourself. Try it again, Mom.

MOTHER (*speaks to Natalie*): So, like when we finished the conversation, and you went back to college, you were left with very difficult and heavy feelings?

NATALIE (*looks at her mother intently, directly into her eyes*): Are you asking?

MOTHER: Yes.

NATALIE (*speaks to her mother*): Are you *really* asking? Really want to know?

MOTHER (*speaks to Natalie*): Yes!

After a long pause, Natalie sighs, and her voice becomes soft and uneven. Her face is clearly sad:

NATALIE: I stopped coming home. I rarely talked to you guys. That's it. It was the worst feeling in the world—to get the message that "you are not part of us, you're not part of the family. We have our family, and you are not part of it." (*Turns to her father*) There was that one time, a little later, that you said to me, "We feel great with Joshua, we feel great with Rebecca, we feel great with Nathan [i.e., all of Natalie's siblings]. . . . The problem is with you." It is like saying, "We are a family with three children, and there is somebody else—me—who is not a part of the family. We can't have her as part of our family because she is a lesbian, and we can't have the other children knowing that she is a lesbian because something terrible will happen." And as long as I can't say it at home, then when I'm home, I am not really there. I feel unwanted (*begins to cry profusely*). I feel like I am alone in the world.

AMPLIFYING VULNERABLE EMOTIONS

This is an important moment in the therapy, when the young adult is able to move from expressing secondary emotions, such as rejecting anger, to accessing more adaptive vulnerable emotions in the presence of their parents. Such shifts make it easier for parents to empathize with their young adult's pain and unmet needs. In the example that follows, Natalie transitions from primarily expressing rejecting anger to accessing and expressing adaptive hurt and deep loneliness and despair. At this moment, the therapist needs to monitor how Natalie's parents are taking in this information—whether it feels like her parents are touched and are softening or whether they are getting defensive:

THERAPIST (*turns to parents*): How are you guys feeling right now?

FATHER: It is upsetting. That is certainly not the message we wanted to send to Natalie. It is not what I meant. . . . I feel regret, a missed opportunity.

THERAPIST: Can you say more?

FATHER: A missed opportunity to continue the conversation, to be there with her in those difficult moments. It makes me sad.

THERAPIST (*speaks to father*): I can see how much you love your daughter— and the sadness in your eyes. Can you check in with Natalie about what she needed from you in those moments? Perhaps what she needs from you right now?

Asking about past or current unmet needs is one of the most effective ways to access, activate, and amplify adaptive emotions (Greenberg, 2012, 2017). The experience of being fully in contact with what one needed or needs in a particular moment and, at the same time, the felt sense of not having those needs met automatically activates adaptive grief and assertive anger.

Adaptive grief is the natural response to the sense of loss associated with what was and no longer exists or what never was. *Assertive anger* is the natural response to recognizing the injustice of not having one's basic, legitimate needs met. Activating and amplifying these adaptive emotions in the room not only help the young adult to better connect to and convey their experience, but also serves as an empathic bridge for parents to connect to their child's emotions and unmet needs:

FATHER (*speaks to Natalie*):   I would be happy to hear. What do you need from me? What would help?

NATALIE (*speaks to her father*):   I just want you to listen. There are things you aren't hearing—like what it is like for me at home not being able to tell my siblings.

FATHER: Okay. What is that like for you?

NATALIE: Do you really want to hear?

FATHER: Yes, I really want to hear.

NATALIE (*Sighs, connecting to her sadness and despair*):   I don't tell my two younger siblings because you two don't want me to. If it were up to me, I would tell them. In the end, it means that they don't really know me or what is going on with me. It is as if I am not really there.

FATHER: Do you feel like it would bring you relief if you could tell them?

This is another critical crossroad in the task. The father, who has begun to connect with his daughter's distress, is instinctively drawn to finding a solution. This is not a bad thing. It is natural and expected. Almost all parents have a hard time seeing their child in pain. Their immediate impulse is to try to solve the problem and reduce their young adult's distress. However, at this point, problem solving is premature. You cannot solve a problem until you fully understand it. Moreover, part of the problem is that the young adult wants to feel heard and understood. Natalie wants her parents to understand what she has been through and how their demand that she conceal her identity has hurt her over the years. Therefore, at this moment in the therapy, the therapist must immediately intervene to block parents' efforts to prematurely fix things. Fixing interrupts exploration. The therapist does this by emphatically assuring family members that there will be a time later in the treatment to think about how to solve problems. The therapist reminds them that, at this point in the therapy, the primary goal is to help them help their young adult to feel fully heard and understood—for her parents to understand deeply what is like for Natalie to have to conceal her identity from her siblings:

THERAPIST (*speaks to father*): Before we get to solutions and how you can make things better for Natalie, I was wondering what you felt inside when you heard Natalie say that?

FATHER: I can totally understand. I can identify with that.

THERAPIST (*speaks to Natalie*): When you hear Dad say that he can identify, how does that feel?

NATALIE: I don't really think he understands.

THERAPIST (*speaks to Natalie*): Can you check in with Dad to see what he understood?

NATALIE (*speaks to her father*): Do you want to tell me what you understood about my feelings?

FATHER (*speaks to Natalie*): Yes. And I have to say, your feelings are very natural. It's clear to me that when there is something significant and core that is being concealed, that is impossible to talk about, it hurts for two reasons. First, like you said, you can't really share things about your life, so it is not really you. You can't bring yourself to the table. Second, when there are family conversations about topics related to sexual orientation, the fact that you can't be open about who you are makes it uncomfortable, embarrassing. That when people ask you things about your future, the fact that you have to hide who you are and avoid answering questions directly is uncomfortable. From all of those directions, I can see how it would be hard, would hurt.

THERAPIST (*speaks to Natalie*): What was that like, hearing Dad's response?

NATALIE (*slowly nods her head and has a subtle smile on her face and a twinge of relief*): Good.

THERAPIST (*speaks to father*): See if Natalie will tell you more about what this has been like for her?

NATALIE: Sure. . . . I feel like it is a big loss for me. That I have missed a couple of years in my relationship with them, my siblings.

THERAPIST (*speaks to mother*): And what is it like for you to hear Natalie say the things she is sharing?

MOTHER: It hurts me to hear her pain. But I am happy that she is sharing this. It is a hard process, but I am glad she is saying all of this.

MEANING MAKING

At the end of this first attachment session, and every subsequent attachment session, the therapist checks in with family members to see how it was for them. This is important. Successful corrective attachment episodes touch on deep, emotion-laden material that has not previously been talked about and processed in such an open, sustained manner. Consequently, these episodes are stirring, evocative, and powerful. The therapist needs to leave enough time at the end of the session to help family members reflect; make meaning of what happened; and, when necessary, to down-regulate and gather themselves. In the following and last segment of this first attachment session, the therapist checks in with both Natalie and her parents:

THERAPIST: How was the conversation for you today?

NATALIE: I think it was an important conversation. I think we are on the right track, but it is hard.

THERAPIST: In what way was it hard?

NATALIE: I think important things were opened up, but this is a safe place. I don't know what it is going to be like the next time I visit at home. I worry that my parents might go back to how it was in the past, argue with me about irrelevant details, and that will be even more hurtful.

THERAPIST (*turns to parents*): What about you two?

FATHER: I also think it was important. This is why we came. We need somebody to help us talk about these things. I think we should put all of this aside between sessions. When we are all home for the weekend, let's not talk about this alone yet. We can all hold on to this optimism that we are working on this finally, and wait until we meet here again.

At this point, the therapist often congratulates family members for the progress they have made. We acknowledge the emotionally challenging nature of the work and recognize family members for their courage and persistence. We also validate family members' fears about what might happen between sessions. For example, Natalie fears that her parents might regress or even seek retribution after the family leaves the room. Parents, for their part, sometimes worry that they will not be able to function in the days following the session. They are afraid that the painful emotions evoked during the session will continue to reverberate and perhaps overwhelm them. The therapist should normalize such fears. We might also need to strategize with family members about how to avoid destructive interactions between sessions that might undermine the work they have begun to do. The therapist can help family members think about how to self-soothe, coregulate, or otherwise help each other if they find themselves feeling overwhelmed or in conflict.

Subsequent attachment sessions are opportunities for family members to raise additional and still unresolved traumatic memories, frustrating and hurtful family dynamics, unmet needs, and associated emotions. For example, in the next attachment session with Natalie and her parents, Natalie decided to share with her parents, for the first time, her experience of feeling alone and abandoned after she and her girlfriend broke up:

THERAPIST: Okay. We are going to continue with the same type of work you all were able to do last week—talk about some of the things that have been hard to talk about in the past. Natalie, there were a couple of other topics you and I spoke about when we met alone. Do you want to choose one of them to start?

NATALIE (*speaks to parents*): So, one of the things I had brought up with [name of therapist] was what happened this past winter. Liz [Natalie's girlfriend] and I separated at the end of the fall, and it was really, really hard for me. It was terrible. And there were 2 or 3 months that you guys didn't know anything about it; you weren't in the picture. She went back to Belgium, and I was just starting college. I was living in a new city with a bunch of new people that I didn't know, and the beginning was hard. And it was really, really horrible because everything happened at the same time. I had to deal with the breakup alone because all my friends were away at different colleges. I saw you guys as like a last resort—a place where I could come and simply feel like everything was going to be all right despite all that I was going through. Yes, it is true that at that point, our relationship already wasn't great. It was complicated for all types of reasons. But I was looking for something that I could hold on to. I felt like I didn't have anybody . . . at all . . . in the whole world. . . . And when I did turn to you, I felt like I got the cold shoulder. I didn't have that place where somebody would say, "Wow! You are dealing with so many things. We are here. We are here to help you. We see you. We see your struggles. We see the things that you are going through" . . . that just wasn't there, and . . . it was like being in a dark hole and reaching out for help and not receiving . . . a hand . . . in return (*long silence ensues*).

THERAPIST (*turns to father*):   I saw you nodding when you heard Natalie speaking.

FATHER: I understand completely the terrible pain she is describing. (*Turns to Natalie*) A breakup is a very difficult thing. I have experienced that myself. And then add to that the fact that you were in a new city. I can only imagine how painful that must have been.

NATALIE: You never said anything like that to me back then. . . .

FATHER: You're right.

NATALIE: You didn't say, "I understand your pain about the breakup." Up until now, I haven't heard anything like that from you.

THERAPIST: What is it like to hear that from Dad right now?

NATALIE: It feels good to hear that (*shows a clear sense of relief*). . . . Yes, it feels good.

THERAPIST (*speaks to father*):   Dad, this is an opportunity for you to go back to that same period, ask some questions, be with her in that experience, at least in retrospect. Be with her and understand what she went through.

FATHER (*turns to Natalie*):   I would be happy to hear more now, if you are willing. I don't want to intrude, but if you are willing, I want to hear.

NATALIE: It was really, really hard (*begins to sob and looks at her father's face*). She flew back to Belgium, and we were still in contact for a while.

FATHER: What did the two of you think would happen? What was the plan?

NATALIE: That I would be here for a year. And that we would be in a long-distance relationship. And after a year, we would be together again. And then, soon after she left, she broke up with me. . . . I didn't want the relationship to end. (*Sobbing increases*) Everything just fell apart.

Later in the session:

NATALIE: I couldn't let anybody know about me. It's like . . . somebody who just broke up with her boyfriend—for example, she can simply talk about it, she can let it out. She can say to people around her, "I just broke up with my boyfriend," and people will look at her with acceptance and understanding. I didn't even have that option! To talk about it with my roommates . . . or at home.

FATHER: Do you still feel it today?

NATALIE: Feel what?

FATHER: The pain you are describing. Or are you already past it?

NATALIE: Less. But it still hurts, but a lot less.

FATHER: And was the pain about the fact that it ended, the loss, or the way that it ended?

NATALIE: Both. It was mixed. I think the bigger part was to lose Liz because she was really important to me. That was the harder part, the part about the loss. Because she filled a very, very big place in my life. We were together 24/7. It was a really intensive relationship. And in a lot of ways, she saved me. When I was with her, I had some of the happiest months of my life. Until it ended. . . . But it was a good relationship. It was a relationship that filled something up inside of me. And suddenly it ended, and the way in which it ended, it was like a crash. And it was extreme. I might have been blind, but I didn't see it coming. I was with her in the summer, and it was like I was on a high, and then when she broke up with me, everything fell apart.

After a long pause and seeing the pain on both of Natalie's parents' faces, the therapist prompts Natalie's parents to respond. Again, the potency of this therapy is in the new relational experiences formed between the young adult and their parents in the session. Unlike individual therapy in which young adults process their emotions alone with the therapist, in ABFT-SGM, the young adult experiences their parents' more attuned, caring, empathic responses in vivo. Such new relational experiences are the primary mechanism of change in ABFT-SGM. Rather than just having family members talk about how to be different, the therapist helps them actually *be* different in the therapy session. This transforms their experience of one another and of the relationship itself:

THERAPIST: What does it do to the two of you to hear Natalie speak like this? Or see her like this?

FATHER: It is very, very sad and painful. The fact that she had to go through this. After all of the other challenges she has had. After the crisis she had with us, and then when it looks like there is a light at the end of the tunnel, she is suddenly hit with something like that. . . . It makes me sad. (*Turns and looks directly at Natalie*) I can only imagine how you felt. That is the last thing in the world that you deserved (*Natalie begins to sob*). Especially after all that you've been through.

MOTHER: It is heartbreaking. I saw you were unhappy, but I had no idea. I wish I had known and could have been there for you.

THERAPIST (*speaks to Natalie*): What's going on with you right now inside, Natalie, when you hear your parents say those things? (*Natalie quietly sobs for a few minutes.*)

In these moments, the therapist waits patiently. Our ability to fearlessly remain present helps parents like Natalie's sit with their young adult's pain. Such moments are powerful and therapeutic. For the first time, Natalie is experiencing this deep pain with her parents by her side rather than alone. Through the process of memory reconsolidation (Nadel et al., 2008), this new experience blends with, and serves to revise, Natalie's past memories of the same event. Now, when her memories of these events are activated, she will feel differently—less alone (Greenberg, 2012). How long to stay in this moment is a clinical decision. The therapist wants the family to remain long enough for the moment to sink in but not so long that it becomes forced or intolerable, or it dissipates. After deciding to move on, the therapist explores how family members hold and comfort one another in such moments of sadness and loss:

THERAPIST (*speaks to parents*): How do you two typically comfort your daughter when you see her this upset?

FATHER: Over the past few years, for all kinds of reasons, we never had conversations like this. There were times in the past that I was with her in difficult times. . . .

NATALIE (*speaks over her father*):   They never see me like this (*becomes more regulated*).

THERAPIST (*speaks to Natalie*):   When Dad said, "I can understand," and Mom said that she wished she had seen and could have been there with you, I saw that it touched you.

NATALIE: I think it freed up something inside of me. Before it was like a war. (*Speaks directly to her parents*) It's nice that you two understand (*smiles gently, sadly*). I am happy that you understand.

In the following attachment session, Natalie and her father process the loss they both experienced as the result of the rupture in their relationship after her coming out. They reminisce about the positive moments and feelings they once shared and disclose how they both long to have that special tie again:

THERAPIST (*speaks to Natalie*):   In one of our sessions alone, you talked about how important your relationship with your father was when you were growing up. You talked about how close the two of you were, and then suddenly, it was like losing something dear. The relationship, his pride in you. . . . You talked about feeling like he now looks at you with a little less admiration and pride. . . .

NATALIE (*turns to speak to her father directly*):   It's like . . . once I was the most wonderful thing in the world to you . . . and I dropped a number of levels in your eyes (*begins to cry*).

THERAPIST (*speaks to father*):   Did you know how important it was to Natalie, your esteem for her, how proud you are of her?

FATHER: It is true that we used to have a wonderful relationship. (*Turns to speak directly to Natalie*) As far as I am concerned, it doesn't have to end. I still love you and admire you to the same degree I always have. I think that what happened between us over the past few years was the result of a bad process. It does not reflect how I feel about you. The way things unfolded was not ideal. I love you like I always have, and you are uniquely special. And my dialogue with you, the conversations we have, are something very meaningful for me.

THERAPIST (*turns to Natalie*):   What is going on inside of you, after hearing Dad say that? Do you believe him? Do you not believe him?

NATALIE: I don't know . . . (*long silence ensues*). (*Turns to speak directly to her father*) I think that what happened, your reaction after I told you that I was lesbian, scared me. To see you act in ways that I had never seen before. I had never seen you angry like that before. . . . I had never seen you scared that way before . . . anxious . . . worried. . . . And I think that is part of it. . . . I saw parts of you that. . . .

FATHER (*nods in acknowledgment*):   Yes, I never saw myself in such a state either (*smiles*).

Father, mother, and Natalie laugh together in acknowledgment. The tension in the room decreases. The therapist speaks to Natalie:

THERAPIST: Now that you hear Dad saying, "Yes. I was in a state of distress that I had never experienced before, but I love and admire you as much as I ever did," how does that make you feel? Do you believe him?

NATALIE: Yes. But I am also afraid to get hurt again (*begins to cry*).

THERAPIST: Afraid to open up again, to be close again . . .? (*Natalie nods "yes," and her crying increases.*) That is something that you want, to feel that again, but it is scary? (*Natalie nods "yes" and continues to cry.*) Could you tell that to Dad right now? That you want to be close again, to open up, but that you are afraid of getting hurt?

NATALIE (*turns to her father*):   I want us to be able to talk. But I am afraid to share something with you and then have you get angry at me or pull away.

FATHER: Again, I think that what happened to us these last few years was a result of a bad process. If we had done something like this [the therapy] before, I don't think we would have reached this point. I think that now that we are talking about all of this openly, we will be in a completely different spot. My love and appreciation of you, Natalie, never waned throughout all of this.

In the preceding example, the therapist helps Natalie share, for the first time, the depth of her disappointment, anger, hurt, fear, and sense of being abandoned. At the same time, the therapist helps her parents put their own feelings aside and invite Natalie to share her feelings more fully than ever before. Their ability to remain steadfastly focused on Natalie's experience, ask for more details, respond in a nondefensive, empathic manner, and validate her feelings was transformative for her. By the end of the task, Natalie clearly felt a sense of relief, more valued, secure, and connected.

Returning to the example of the Levy family first introduced in Chapter 5, the son Alex is less concerned about being hurt and invalidated. Instead, he worries about causing his mother pain. He describes being torn between wanting to be more open with his parents and his concern about causing his mother more distress. His mother, on the other hand, says she wants to be closer to her son, to know more about the details of his life and what he has been through over the years. At the same time, she is terrified about being overwhelmed with feelings of guilt, pain, hopelessness, and shame.

In the segment that follows, the therapist begins the attachment task with the Levy family by marking the goal of the task and explicitly acknowledging family members' fears and ambivalence. When families are apprehensive, we often begin by "talking about talking" rather than just jumping into the thick of things. We first talk about their concerns about opening up and their fears about what might happen. Then, we assure them that we will go at their pace and support them as necessary. The therapist is confident. They believe in the importance of the work, in family member's inner resources, and in their own ability to recognize when and how to adjust the therapy in a way that family members do not get hurt and the process is productive:

THERAPIST: So, we have made it to this day. You folks are all ready. This is an opportunity for you to talk about important things that have been hard to talk about up until now. But I know that you have some concerns, fears about having these conversations. Can we start with that?

MOTHER: I am the kind of person who has a hard time hearing painful things. But we are doing this with our eyes open and know that it may be hard. We have reached the point where we have to open things up. I know it.

THERAPIST (*speaks to Alex*):   I know that you are worried about your mom. That you are concerned that if you are more open with her, are more direct, it will cause her too much pain.

ALEX: I do worry about that. That is constantly in my mind. It influences my behavior. On the other hand, the alternative of not talking about how I feel, not telling . . . has become too painful.

I also think that in the end, telling them [his parents] more about myself will actually make them feel better.

MOTHER: I know that I want to do this. It is just hard for me to get started—to take that first step.

This is a beautiful moment of honesty and vulnerability on the mother's part. She takes responsibility for who she is—her strengths and weaknesses—rather than trying to make her son feel guilty. But she also gives her son permission to be honest, to put his needs above hers and not worry about taking care of her. The mother's clear and courageous stance that she wants to hear more at all costs allows Alex to take the next step:

THERAPIST (*speaks to both Alex and his mother*): Okay. This is the place to do it. Even though this is hard for you, I know that you are capable and want to have this conversation. I am also here to help and support both of you. Why don't you give it a try now?

ALEX: Try what?

MOTHER (*speaks to Alex*): To tell us about all of those things that you went through in the past but had to keep secret—that you couldn't tell us about.

ALEX: Okay.

MOTHER (*pauses, then speaks to Alex*): I know that in order to move forward, we need to open things up. I know that it will be hard for me, but I know that this is what we have to do.

THERAPIST: Okay. Let's try to do it step by step. (*Speaks to mother*) When we met alone last week, you mentioned a couple of things that you thought were important and that you had never asked Alex about directly. Now you have the chance to do that—to invite him to share those things with the two of you.

MOTHER (*turns to Alex with an empathic but pained face*): The first thing I wanted to ask was. . . . Ethan's mother [the mother of one of Alex's friends] told me that he told her that he was gay when he was 14. You only told us a few years ago, when you were 22. I imagine you had known for many years. How come you didn't tell us earlier? More importantly, how did you cope with it all of those years without telling us? I imagine that now, at this age, being older, it is easier to deal with. But as a youngster, a teenager, I imagine it was hard to deal with.

ALEX: Actually, I was lucky. I had a bunch of friends who all came out, each in their own time. We felt like we had a tight-knit group of good friends. It was me, Dana, Liam, Eli, and Anna. I had a good experience in high school. We stuck together.

MOTHER: Did you ever get teased or harassed? How did other kids in your class react?

ALEX: I was actually one of the more popular kids in the school. Everybody knew that I was gay, but, for the most part, it was a nonissue. I got along with everybody. I think that people treated me that way because I accepted myself. I was confident and didn't hide who I was.

FATHER: What about in the army? Did people know? Were you harassed or called things like "homo"?

ALEX: Even in my combat unit, people knew. Because I accepted it as natural and not as a big thing, they did, too. People would ask me questions, they were interested. Last year, my commanding officer, who I hadn't seen in 7 years, invited me and Dan [Alex's partner] to his wedding. Everybody was so excited and happy to see me and meet Dan. It is a nonissue with them. I am very loved and accepted.

THERAPIST (*checks in with parents*):   How is it for the two of you to hear these things? I know that this is new information.

FATHER: It makes me happy. I feel relieved.

THERAPIST (*turns to mother*):   And you?

MOTHER: It feels good. I also feel some relief.

At this point, the mother returns to focusing on the rupture in her and her husband's relationship with Alex:

MOTHER: And you didn't feel like you could tell us?

ALEX: I didn't want to hurt you. I knew how hard you would take it. I know how important it is for you that everything is perfect, by the book. I know how you worry about things.

THERAPIST (*speaks to mother, who begins to cry*):   I see that this is bringing up strong feelings for you. Can you say what you are feeling?

MOTHER: It makes me sad—that he didn't feel like I was strong enough for him to confide in me.

THERAPIST (*speaks to mother*): And that is something that you would want? For him to feel like you are strong enough for him to be more open with you? To be able to be there with him and know what is going on in his life?

MOTHER: Of course. With all of the pain, what kind of relationship is it if we aren't open with each other?

Later in the session, Alex's father shifts to asking Alex questions about his sexual identity development. This line of questioning is actually quite common among the parents ABFT-SGM therapists see. Because children with nonaccepting parents tend to conceal so much from their parents, their parents typically have little knowledge of the process their child has gone through over the years and the experiences that have shaped their child's sexual identity development. This leaves parents with fragmented and sometimes seemingly conflicting pieces of information. This can be confusing and anxiety producing for parents.

In contrast, when parents have more complete knowledge about their child's identity development, they have an easier time putting the pieces together. They can form a more coherent narrative, allowing them to fully see and accept their child for who they are. Therefore, as long as parents are asking questions in an open, curious manner, are not being intrusive, are not trying to challenge or disconfirm their young adult's experience, and as long as the young adult feels comfortable answering their parents' questions, such conversations are productive and important:

FATHER: You just mentioned that almost all of the friends of yours that I know are gay. I wonder if you felt like, maybe with all of them coming out, that you got sucked into it?

ALEX (*laughs*): No. Not at all.

FATHER: From what age did you feel like you were attracted to boys and not girls?

ALEX: From elementary school. From the age of 11 or 12.

FATHER (*shows surprise but in an open, curious manner*): From that early an age, you already knew that you were gay?

ALEX: Not that I was gay but who I found myself looking at. Who I was interested in. Even then, I knew. But I was fine with that.

It's not like it was "cool" or "in." Even in Israel, in 2022, I still can't get married, still can't have a child through surrogacy. There is nothing "easy" or "cool" to get sucked into.

FATHER: Did you ever, at any point, try to be with women?

ALEX: No.

FATHER (*shows surprise, looks a bit hurt*): That is not what you told me when I asked you when you were hanging out with that girl in 12th grade. You told me that the two of you were boyfriend and girlfriend.

ALEX (*is a bit embarrassed*): That was the one time I lied to you about it. You surprised me with the question. I had to react fast, and I am sorry. But I assure you, I was never with a woman.

FATHER (*looks disappointed*): It never crossed your mind? How can you be absolutely sure that you are not attracted to women if you have never been with one?

ALEX: Have you ever been with men? Did you ever try?

FATHER: No.

ALEX: Why not?

FATHER: Because I have no attraction to them, and it isn't natural.

ALEX: That is exactly how it is for me. I have no attraction to them and it isn't natural. I know who I am, how I feel. I have a partner I love for the past 4½ years. Some people live their whole lives and never have the fortune of having the type of love I have. I could be sitting here, straight, at the age of 30, with nobody special in my life. I am happy with who I am, where I am at, and what my life is like. My life is great. I want you to be happy with me, for me.

A little later in the session, Alex's father asks him who else in the family knows about his sexual orientation. This is a common concern of parents. It stems from parents' shame and fear regarding how others will react. Such conversations are important because, almost inevitably, parents learn that more people actually know than they had imagined. These conversations are also important because parents typically hear that other people's responses were more positive than parents had feared. Such conversations serve as a form of indirect or vicarious exposure. Hearing that others responded positively decreases parents' fear, leads to relief, and can engender motivation and courage to take the next step in their own coming out process. Parents' own coming out, in turn, facilitates further acceptance of their young adult's sexual or gender identity. Likewise, parents' increased acceptance makes it easier for them to be open with others. Indeed, parental acceptance is strongly correlated with parents' level of disclosure and with positive responses from family, friends, and community members:

FATHER: Who in the extended family knows? Which of your aunts and cousins?

ALEX: Shirley, Micah, Jordan. . . . Basically, everybody knows.

FATHER (*shows surprise*): And how did everybody react?

ALEX: I was over at Uncle Simon's house for dinner last week with Dan, and Aunt Lilly happened to call. When she heard that Dan and I were there, she asked me to pick up the phone and then told me they were angry at me that I hadn't told them earlier. They said that they want to have Dan and me over so that they can meet him as soon as possible. Others called just to say that they heard, and they wanted me to know that they were happy for me.

THERAPIST: I want to pause for a second and just check in with the two of you (*looks at parents*) to hear how you are feeling right now with all of this new information.

FATHER: Naturally, one's biggest fears are about the unknown—how people are going to react, what they are going to say. And the more that the unknown becomes known, you become less afraid. You don't have any worries anymore! You don't have to keep it secret!

THERAPIST: So, there is some relief?

FATHER: A lot of relief. . . .

These types of conversations in which parents ask questions about things they never dared to ask about before are important on a number of levels. First, the information they gain helps them form a more complete and coherent narrative of the past. They suddenly understand their child's behaviors and past events in a different way. Things that were confusing before suddenly make sense. Second, there is something powerful and freeing about finally speaking openly and honestly about things that have been kept hidden for years. At the end of such conversations, parents and their young adult typically feel some sense of relief. Third, the information parents gain can serve to decrease their anxiety about the future. When they hear that their child has a partner, is happy, that people treat them well at work, that they have a strong support and friend network of people who know they are lesbian, gay, bisexual, transgender, or queer, parents can relax somewhat. Some of the catastrophic fears that they have carried around for years dissipate. Aside from relief, hearing about their young adult's initiative, resilience, successes, and happiness also often elicits feelings of joy, pride, and hope.

The next and final example is taken from work with the Robinson family. Shai, age 27, had brought his mother to therapy because he felt like she was having a hard time accepting his transition from female to male. He was both worried about her but also frustrated. He felt like her lack of understanding, anxiety, and slow progress in accepting his trans identity was thwarting his ability to move forward with exploring and performing his gender in a free, authentic manner.

Over the course of the attachment task, Shai and his mother, Claire, had a number of meaningful, productive conversations. They talked openly about Shai's experience of his gender, about his desire to present to the world in a more typically masculine manner, and about his future plans to have gender affirming surgery. As the treatment progressed, Shai became increasingly forthcoming and honest with his mother, and his mother showed incredible strength, courage, and caring. She asked questions; empathized with Shai's feelings and needs; attended support groups; and was genuine about her own confusion, grief, and anxiety. Throughout the process, however, she consistently made it clear that her number one priority was that Shai be happy. She was committed to becoming more comfortable with and supportive of his gender identity—even if the road was still hard for her.

The following segment, taken from their last attachment session, illustrates how the therapist helped Shai and Claire use the attachment task to the fullest. After congratulating them on the meaningful progress they had made thus far, and before bringing the task to an end, the therapist explored whether there were any remaining important topics that they wanted to broach. The trust, safety, and intimacy that develops over the course of the attachment task creates a unique space in which family members can talk about things that they may never talk about again. The therapist offers this last attachment session as an opportunity to dive deeper, to take yet another chance before moving onto the next and last phase of the treatment:

THERAPIST: You know, the two of you have made extraordinary progress. I wonder how you are both feeling at this point.

MOTHER: I think I am feeling more at ease with this all, with Shai's identity.

SHAI (*turns to his mother*): Mom, you are doing an amazing job, and I really appreciate it.

THERAPIST: Claire, perhaps you could find out from Shai if there are still things that you could do to make him feel even more comfortable when at home with you?

MOTHER (*turns to Shai*): Are there other things that I could do to make you feel more comfortable? Things that I could do or say? Things that still bother you?

SHAI (*speaks hesitantly*): Ugh, I don't know.

THERAPIST (*speaks to Shai*): You know, Shai, this is a wonderful opportunity. Mom is really stepping up. She is saying that she wants to hear more and that she can take it.

SHAI: I know. I really appreciate that.

THERAPIST (*speaks to Shai*): Are you afraid of hurting her feelings or perhaps asking too much from her?

MOTHER (*speaks to Shai*): That is why I am here. We are here so that I can know these things. I can't know what bothers you and what you would like to have change if you don't tell me.

THERAPIST (*speaks to mother*): So, you are saying to Shai that you are strong enough to take it? That you want to hear?

MOTHER (*speaks directly to Shai*): Absolutely. That is why I am here! I am here to learn.

THERAPIST (*speaks to Shai*): You want to give it a try?

SHAI (*speaks to his mother*): One of the things that I worry about is your reaction to hearing my voice.

MOTHER: What do you mean?

SHAI: I know that it bothers you when you hear my deeper voice.

MOTHER: Really?

SHAI: Yes! Don't you remember? A couple of times, you told me to speak higher.

MOTHER: That was a long time ago.

SHAI: Yes, but I still remember. That stayed with me.

MOTHER: I don't think I have noticed your voice being any deeper or said anything about your voice in over a year.

SHAI (*says emphatically*): That is because I try to speak higher whenever I am at home. It is hard. My voice has become deeper because of the hormones. I like my voice the way it is now. But at home with you, I am constantly monitoring the pitch. I don't want to disappoint or annoy you. It just creates stress for me. I understand that it is hard for you, and I don't want . . .

THERAPIST: Hold on for a second, Shai. (*Turns to mother*) Claire, what is going on inside of you as you hear Shai say what he is saying.

MOTHER: I don't want that. The last thing I want is to cause him more stress. He has enough on his plate. (*Speaks to Shai*) I want you to speak with your natural voice, your current voice.

SHAI: It's scary to do that.

MOTHER: Why is it so scary for you?

SHAI: Because I am afraid you will be horrified. Even now that we are talking about it.

MOTHER: I can hear that your voice is lower than it used to be. I am not horrified. You are connected to me. I won't be horrified by anything you do.

SHAI: So, what does it do to you? Does it bother you?

MOTHER: No. I am getting used to it. It's a process, which I am happy to embrace.

SHAI: I am getting used to you getting used to it. For me, it's taking a risk to let you hear my real voice. I am afraid that you might be freaked out and ask me to go back to using a higher voice. That would be devastating.

MOTHER (*speaks to Shai*): I can understand that, but that is not going to happen. I want you to feel like you can be you, without feeling like you are doing something wrong. It doesn't bother me. Are you trying to adjust your voice right now? In this conversation?

SHAI: Yes.

MOTHER: Even now, listening to you, your voice is much lower than mine. It never was before. But it is important for me to stretch my comfort zone, and it is better for you if you know that I am getting used to it.

SHAI: I wish!

MOTHER: Right now, it is about me doing the changes. I am happy to make those changes because I am in a position now—physically and emotionally—that I can do that. And I think it is the right time to take the advantage of that.

THERAPIST (*speaks to Shai*):   Can you let your mother hear what your voice sounds like without making an effort to change its pitch?

SHAI: It's hard. I am so used to trying to speak in a higher octave around her.

MOTHER: Give me a try. If it is too hard for me, I will tell you.

SHAI: It is hard to just let go. Here (*speaks using a lower tone*). . . . This is closer to what my voice is like now.

MOTHER: I have no problem with that. For me, it is barely audible, and I have a good ear for pitch.

THERAPIST (*speaks to mother*):   So, are you saying that you are fine with Shai speaking with his natural voice right now? That you don't want him to stress anymore about trying to change it for you?

MOTHER: Absolutely. (*Turns to Shai*) I want you to stop trying to change your voice for me.

SHAI (*speaks to his mother*):   Thank you. I appreciate that.

THERAPIST (*speaks to Shai*):   How does that feel hearing Mom say that, hearing Mom react that way? Do you believe her? Do you trust her when she says that she is fine with your voice the way it is now?

SHAI: I do. It is a big relief. I just don't know if I will be to let go all at once. I have been doing this for a long time. Now I have to get used to letting go.

Toward the end of this task, the therapist and family members feel the energy level shift as the most pressing, feared, and salient unresolved issues and emotions have been broached and at least partially resolved. Tension decreases, and there is a more flowing, natural quality to the conversation. Family members feel more comfortable raising previously avoided topics. The relationship has become unblocked. There is a collaborative, loving atmosphere and sense that everybody is working together to make the relationship better. This provides a natural segue into the next and final task of the treatment: collaborative planning for the future.

7 CONSOLIDATION OF GAINS AND COLLABORATIVE PLANNING FOR THE FUTURE

The fifth and final task of the treatment involves helping family members consolidate the gains they made over the course of therapy and, together, envision and plan for the future. This task is the natural next step after family members have worked through the core conflicts and relational injuries that had undermined their relationship. By this stage of the treatment, parents are committed to, and actively working toward, being more accepting and affirming of their child's minority identity. Although they may still bear some degree of shame, fear, and loss associated with their young adult's identification as lesbian, gay, bisexual, transgender, or queer, those feelings no longer overwhelm them or dictate how they behave. Tension in their relationship with their young adult has decreased, goodwill and good intentions prevail, and there is a newfound feeling of closeness and hopefulness. In some families, by this stage in the therapy parents have already taken dramatic steps, including meeting their young adult's partner and friends for the first time; coming out to their own family and friends; and standing up in the face of heterosexist, homo(trans)phobic comments or various forms of discrimination. Family members have a sense that they are working together toward a shared goal.

https://doi.org/10.1037/0000352-007
Attachment-Based Family Therapy for Sexual and Gender Minority Young Adults and Their Nonaccepting Parents, by G. M. Diamond and R. Boruchovitz-Zamir
Copyright © 2023 by the American Psychological Association. All rights reserved.

FIGURE 7.1. Structure of the Consolidation of Gains and Collaborative Planning for the Future Task

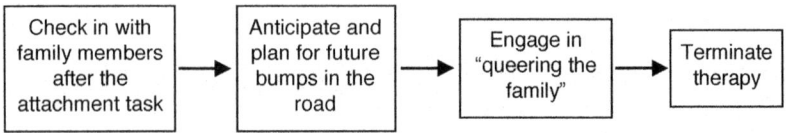

At the start of this task, the therapist checks in with family members regarding how they have been doing since the end of the attachment task (see Figure 7.1). When the therapy has gone well, their responses can be extremely moving. We often hear family members say things like, "We feel like we finally have our son back," "We can talk about things we couldn't talk about before," or "I feel like I am part of the family again." In other cases, family members report more modest gains. For example, one father responded by saying,

> I still have a hard time watching two men hold hands or kiss. I don't think that will ever change. If I had my choice, I would still want my son to be straight. I think that is only natural. Any parent who tells you otherwise is lying. But I do feel much more comfortable about it all. I feel like we can talk openly. I am not ashamed anymore. I don't really care what others think, and I don't hide it from anybody. I also love my son's partner. He is great. He has become part of our family.

Importantly, what may appear to the therapist to be small changes or less than full acceptance can mean the world to the young adult. Families begin treatment at different points on the acceptance continuum and with different expectations. Even small shifts in parents' level of acceptance and family dynamics can be experienced by the young adult as dramatic and meaningful. As therapists, we join family members in celebrating their sense of relief, hopefulness, joy, and renewed connection. We help them to explicitly articulate and take ownership of the important things they did to make these changes possible. We mirror their feelings of accomplishment and pride and admire the courage they showed both within sessions and outside of the therapy room.

ANTICIPATING AND PLANNING FOR FUTURE BUMPS IN THE ROAD

After helping family members consolidate their gains, the focus shifts to helping them identify and plan for potential bumps in the road. Family members know what types of interactions, topics, and situations have been flash points for them in the past. This task is geared to helping them anticipate these situations and strategize how to navigate them if and when they arise. The goal is to prepare family members so that they do not slip back into old negative, destructive relational patterns. During this process, family members imagine what might go wrong and collaboratively problem solve how to respond optimally. This is much easier to do in the therapy room before the event actually occurs rather than in the heat of the moment.

The example that follows was taken from the Cohen family, first introduced in Chapter 3. In this segment, the family begins this task by reveling in Natalie's newfound closeness with her siblings. At the start of treatment, one of Natalie's primary complaints had been that she could not disclose her identity to her younger siblings because of her parents' insistence that she keep her sexual orientation a secret. She felt that her inability to share this personal, essential information with her sister had led to a rupture in their relationship. She lamented that she had once been very close with this same sister and that this secret had torn them apart.

Over the course of the attachment task, her parents were able to hear and understand the destructive effect that their insistence on secrecy had on Natalie and on her relationship with her sister. Consequently, they relented. In coordination with her parents, Natalie finally disclosed to her siblings that she was lesbian.

At the start of this fifth and final task, Natalie recounts an event from the past week illustrating how the process of coming out to her siblings had led to meaningful changes in her relationships with them. Importantly, her parents also expressed their joy and relief to see their children close once again:

FATHER: We had a big surprise when we got back from visiting relatives up north. All of the children were waiting for us at home. They had come from all over the country to greet us.

THERAPIST: Wow! Who organized that?

NATALIE: Rebecca [Natalie's sister]. It was really cool. She thought, "Wouldn't it be fun if we all were waiting for them when they got back." It was great. We sat together waiting, just the four of us, and we just talked. It was great.

THERAPIST: What did you talk about?

NATALIE: All kinds of things. It has been years . . . over 4 years since we have all been together and talked. And it was amazingly natural, easy. It was really great.

THERAPIST: That sounds wonderful. I remember at the beginning of the treatment that was a big thing for you. I remember you talking about how much you missed that closeness and wished it could be different.

NATALIE (*says excitedly*):   Yes. And while we were sitting there, we had some meaningful conversations, sharing in a way I don't remember us talking over the past few years. My brother told me what was going on with him in his new job, and my sister consulted with me about personal stuff that was going on in her life. It was really nice.

THERAPIST (*speaks to parents*):   I imagine that for you two, that is also a good feeling—seeing your children close again.

FATHER: We were in shock. I didn't think I would ever see that day. We prayed for it, hoped for it, but it came all of a sudden.

THERAPIST: It feels like something has shifted. Less tension, more openness, more closeness in the family—that it is easier to talk about stuff.

After reveling in the significant gains that they had made as a family and how much better they all felt, Natalie's father brought up his anxiety about potential future conflicts. He expressed his fear that if, at some point, he felt the need to approach Natalie about something that was bothering him, or she wanted to approach him about something that was bothering her, such conversations might escalate and devolve into an argument. He expressed a wish to find a system for them to be able to have such conversations without it leading to conflict:

FATHER (*speaks to Natalie*):   One thing I would be happy to do is to find some type of mechanism, some way so that if there are specific things that bother you about what I do, or bother me about what you do, we could raise those issues, talk about those things, without it getting misinterpreted and escalating.

NATALIE: I feel like when I come to you and I am upset or angry about something, you immediately take it personally.

THERAPIST: Can you give an example?

NATALIE (*speaks to therapist*):   We recently had an incident where I asked my parents not to do something, and they did it anyway. I told my dad that it really made me angry that they did it, even though I asked them not to. He said, "I don't know what you are angry about. It was all done in good nature. We didn't mean anything bad by it."

THERAPIST (*speaks to father*): Is that how you remember it happening?

FATHER: Yes.

THERAPIST: So, Natalie came to you and told you that she was angry—that she had asked you not to do something, and you did it anyway. And then you responded by explaining to her why she didn't need to be angry.

FATHER: Yes.

THERAPIST (*speaks to Natalie*): Can you tell your father how his response made you feel and how you need him to respond in such instances?

NATALIE (*turns to her father*): I need you to not get defensive. Maybe say, "Really? I didn't realize. I'm sorry. Let me explain my side because I didn't mean to hurt you, but I would like to hear more about why it made you angry."

THERAPIST (*speaks to father*): How does that sound, what Natalie is saying?

FATHER: It is hard to put my finger on the exact moment that . . . when somehow it becomes so loaded, so explosive. In general, the type of person I am . . . when there is a conflict with somebody, I try to speak in a regulated, calm manner. In general, it is hard for me when things escalate and yelling begins.

THERAPIST: And when Natalie comes to you in a state of anger, what happens to you in that moment?

FATHER: My first response is, "Why are you so angry? There is no reason to be that angry. Nobody intentionally meant to do anything wrong. Let's try to understand what the problem is."

THERAPIST: So, your first impulse is to try to kind of calm things down. To deescalate things.

FATHER: Yes. That is what I do in all aspects of my life.

THERAPIST (*speaks to Natalie*): And that is exactly what annoys you. Like he is saying, "You are exaggerating. Things are not the way you think. You are angry for no good reason"?

NATALIE: To say the sentence, "What is there to be angry about?" feels like he is saying my feelings are unjustified.

THERAPIST (*speaks to Natalie*):   And what would be a better response for you in those moments?

NATALIE: If he were to say, "Wait a minute. What is going on that is making you so angry? Let's take a deep breath and calm down, but I want to hear why you are so upset."

FATHER (*speaks to Natalie*):   I can understand how that would be a better response. But it is something that I need to practice. . . . But it needs to go both ways. (*Turns to therapist*) When we, Sarah [his wife] and I, are angry with Natalie, we need to know that we can approach her without it leading to an explosion.

NATALIE: I am willing to hear the things that bother you. But you have to understand that when you tell me that something is bothering you about me, it sits on a long history of me feeling like you are minimizing my feelings and that you are disappointed in me because I am lesbian.

FATHER: I understand. It doesn't come from there, but I understand that any criticism or anger is particularly sensitive because of the past.

THERAPIST (*speaks to father*):   I think it is a big challenge. How to set limits and express anger, while at the same time giving Natalie the message that it is not about who she is as a person or about her sexual orientation.

In the next session, a week later, the therapist checks in with family members about how they felt after the previous session:

THERAPIST: How are you folks?

FATHER (*All three family members smile and nod in the affirmative*):   Things are good. We have been together for the past 2 weeks, and there have been no dramas.

THERAPIST: How did you all feel after the last session?

NATALIE: Good. (*Turns to her father*) It was important for me to hear what you said in the last session. It helped me to better understand where you are coming from. That the moment that I come to you in a state of anger and I am worked up, it automatically makes you step back and tell me that I can't talk to you that way. That your first instinct is to say, "First, let's calm down." And that your way of responding is not just in relation to me.

FATHER: It is something I learned a long time ago from a wise rabbi. He said to me, "The moment you answer somebody in anger, you have already lost." I think that is a really important lesson. When somebody comes at you in a state of agitation, and they are aroused and aggressive, if you respond by putting out your hands in a manner meant to tell them to calm down. . . .

NATALIE: I understand. But in the past, I interpreted it as you saying, "I am not going to pay attention to your anger, to how you are feeling." Like, when I come to you upset, even yelling, and you respond in a calm, detached way, it feels like you are saying, "I am not interested that you are angry."

FATHER (*nods affirmatively, a little embarrassed*): Okay. . . . That is important to know. Sometimes it is important to hear the other side, how things are received. So, for you, it feels like indifference? (*Natalie and her mother nod affirmatively.*)

NATALIE (*explains to therapist*): When we talked last week, I realized that when somebody comes to him [her father] really angry and aggressively, he is not able to speak in that state. That first he needs things to be calmer. In that state, he can't hear or be interested in what the other is thinking or feeling. I suddenly understood that. Before I thought that when he didn't respond, it meant he simply didn't care.

FATHER: I don't always succeed in communicating what I really mean.

NATALIE: My only request is that you don't say to me, "Don't be angry." Say to me, "I want to hear what you have to say, but let's do it in a calmer way."

FATHER: All right. That is important for me to hear.

Later in the session:

NATALIE (*speaks to her father*): When you get angry at me, it takes on extra dimensions. It is not only what I did or what is happening in the moment. When I see your anger, it connects with my feeling that you are angry at me generally for who I am, the person I have become. That's why it is so hard for me. When

> I hear your criticism, I carry it around in me for weeks. It hits me in the core. It feels like you are critical, disappointed in me being lesbian.

The preceding example illustrates how family members work together to better understand each other's states of mind, their intentions, what happens to each of them during certain types of interactions, what core issues are activated, and how to adjust their responses accordingly. They understand how the other interprets and experiences their words and behaviors. They also become privy to the fears, sensitivities, and vulnerabilities of each other as well what each of them needs to feel safe, heard, and respected.

Unlike earlier stages of the treatment, when the focus of the therapy is primarily on the young adult's experience and needs, during this task, the focus is more balanced. Parents have more of a chance to talk about themselves and their own experience. Because during the attachment task, the young adult finally feels heard, at this point in the treatment, parents' self-disclosure is not experienced as defensiveness. It is not perceived as an attempt by parents to justify their behavior, make excuses, or blame. Consequently, the young adult is open to listening. This allows the young adult to learn new things about their parents—things that they did not know or understand before. This typically leads them to see their parents in a more complete and complex manner, and through more compassionate eyes. This, in turn, promotes magnanimity. Family members begin to work more collaboratively. They are committed to finding ways to meet each other's needs in future encounters so as to avoid destructive interactions and improve the relationship.

QUEERING THE FAMILY

Another goal of this fifth and final task is what Stone Fish and Harvey (2005) termed *queering the family*, which refers to the process of not only normalizing and accepting the young adult's sexual orientation or gender identity but also affirming, embracing, and nurturing it, both within the family of origin and vis-à-vis others. For example, during this task, family members often strategize how and when to disclose the young adult's sexual orientation or gender identity to family members and friends who still do not know, and how to welcome their young adult's partner into the family. Parents explore how to become more involved in their young adult's life, learn more about their young adult's experience of being who they are and the world they live in, and explore how they can become better advocates for their young adult and the lesbian, gay, bisexual, transgender, and queer (LGBTQ+) community in general.

In a later segment with the Cohen family, Natalie and her parents thought together about how and when to come out to her grandparents. Before the start of treatment, Natalie's parents had been resistant to the idea of her coming out to her grandparents. They feared that it might make her grandparents sad and anxious and that they would have to contain and soothe their grandparents' shame and fear. Moreover, they were concerned that such a disclosure would negatively affect how her grandparents perceived Natalie. They described how her grandparents had always held Natalie in high esteem, and they were afraid that Natalie would lose that.

Over the course of treatment, Natalie conveyed to her parents how important it was for her to be authentic and open with her grandparents, whom she respected and loved dearly. Consequently, her parents agreed to help her plan the best way to go about telling them:

MOTHER: What were you thinking in terms of when and how to tell them?

NATALIE: I don't know. I just kind of thought I would go over to see them on Sunday evening like I usually do. That I would just tell them that I have a girlfriend. That I am not interested in men. That it was important for me that they know because we have such a close relationship. What do you two think?

FATHER (*looks nervous*): Are you planning to tell them both at the same time?

NATALIE: I hadn't really thought about it. Why?

FATHER: I just wonder if it might not be better to tell Pop-pop first.

MOTHER: Pop-pop is a much more open, easygoing person than Mum-mum. I don't think it is going to shake him. I think he is going to be fine from the start. He also knows how to handle Mum-mum, communicate things to her at the right time and with the right words so that they kind of land right.

NATALIE: I am fine with that, if you think that will be better.

FATHER: In any event, we are all going to be together next Wednesday for Rebecca's birthday.

MOTHER: That is not a problem. I am sure Pop-pop will tell Mum-mum by then, and then (*turns to Natalie*) you can approach Mum-mum

154 •   *Attachment-Based Family Therapy for Sexual and Gender Minority Young Adults*

> directly if you want. I think it will just give her a couple of days
> to kind of process it before the two of you talk directly.

THERAPIST (*speaks to mother*):   Can you check in with Natalie to see how
she feels about that plan.

MOTHER (*speaks to Natalie*):   Does that sound like a reasonable plan? Are
you agreeable to telling Pop-pop first and then waiting a day
before telling Mum-mum?

NATALIE: I agree. Sometimes Mum-mum does need a day or so to digest
things; otherwise, she just kinds of shuts down. I think it is
a good plan. After all of these years, I don't mind waiting
another couple of days before she knows (*smiles*).

The following segment, taken from the Green family, is another example
of how families use the last sessions to collaboratively problem solve and
plan for the future. Noah, aged 30, identified as nonbinary and preferred
to be addressed using female pronouns. She had identified publicly as male
for most of her life and, at the start of therapy, had not yet come out to her
extended family or asked them to change their manner of addressing her.

During the attachment task, she was able to convey to her parents her
experience of feeling neither completely male nor completely female. She
also explained how aversive it felt when people addressed her using male
pronouns and how natural and affirming it felt when they addressed her
using female pronouns. Consequently, her parents agreed to help her more
fully express her gender identity in social settings, including at gatherings of
the extended family. At the same time, they were afraid of how others would
react, worried that Noah would be ridiculed or shunned. The following
segment illustrates how family members worked together in an effort to
help Noah live as authentically and openly as possible:

NOAH: I don't feel comfortable coming to family events dressed as a
man and hearing people address me in the masculine.

FATHER: So, what do you want to do about it?

NOAH: I want to ask people to use female pronouns when speaking to
me. I want to dress in a way that makes me feel good.

MOTHER: Do you have an idea of what you want to wear?

NOAH: I am not sure yet. I am still figuring it out. I think I would
prefer wearing one of the flowing shirts that I have. I also want
to wear nail polish and a necklace.

FATHER (*speaks in a concerned, nonjudgmental tone*): Are you worried about how some of the family might react?

NOAH: To be honest, I am not that worried. I know that my cousins will be fine. And I know how to take Uncle Alan's comments with a grain of salt, how to ignore him. Even if I just hang out with the few people who I know, I will be fine with that. At least I will feel comfortable with myself. That is better than continuing to feel like I am wearing a mask, not being myself.

MOTHER: What would you like us to say to people if they ask us why you are dressed that way?

FATHER (*speaks to mother*): What are you worried about? We will tell them the truth—that Noah prefers that people turn to him (*quickly corrects himself*) to *her* using female pronouns. That she feels more like a woman than a man and that is just the way it is. If they have more questions about it, they can ask Noah directly.

MOTHER (*speaks to Noah*): Is that the way you want us to handle it?

NOAH: I think that is the best approach. The two of you do not need to explain for me. If people want to ask me about my gender, they can ask me directly. I am happy to talk to them about it.

The third example is taken from the Gold family, first introduced in Chapter 3. In the segment that follows, Adam and his parents begin this fifth task noting the progress that father has made in terms of accepting Adam being gay, as well as the work that still needs to be done. As the conversation progresses, Adam's father talks about how he has come out to his circle of closest friends. He also talks about his desire to become a stronger advocate for his son's civil rights and the rights of all LGBTQ+ people:

FATHER: We had a good weekend. I stood by my commitment and completed my homework.

ADAM (*smiles, speaks to his father*): I didn't even know that you had homework.

FATHER: Yes, I was supposed to tell our group of friends. We had a social evening. Somebody came and brought these cards, and we were all supposed to talk about something that other people didn't know about us, also about our dreams for the future. . . .

MOTHER: He slipped it in the middle of talking about the family as a whole.

FATHER: I usually hide behind Ruth [his wife]. I let her tell things. This time, I initiated.

ADAM: And do you feel better, relieved that they now know?

FATHER: When I told my boss last week, I felt relief. This time, I didn't have that same feeling.

ADAM: But did it make you feel worse?

FATHER: No. It didn't really have an impact. Maybe because it is not the first time. Maybe because there was such a sense of relief after telling my boss, it's not as new or stressful anymore.

MOTHER: He did a great job. I was watching him from the side. Afterwards, he got a hug and kiss from me.

FATHER (*speaks to his wife*): And how did you feel when I told everybody?

MOTHER: I felt fine. I didn't have a problem with it in the first place. My only problem was that *you* were not ready to tell people.

FATHER: It also made me feel like I wanted to go to the demonstration that is planned in Tel Aviv in support of surrogacy for gay couples. (*Turns to his wife*) I wrote Adam a text saying that I wanted to go.

MOTHER (*sounds surprised and happy*): Really?! (*Turns to Adam*) He wrote you a text saying that he wanted to go to the demonstration?

ADAM (*smiles*): Yes.

MOTHER (*still smiling*): Wow!

FATHER: I have no problem going to that demonstration. I want to go. It is not the same as the Pride parade. There is nothing provocative about it. Here, there is a specific, important issue at hand.

ADAM: And do you identify with the cause? The rights of gays to use surrogacy?

FATHER: I do.

ADAM: But that runs counter to what you said before. You said you were not sure you would be able to accept it if I wanted to bring kids into the world.

FATHER: I think that because of these sessions, I have made a few steps— maybe not giant steps, but my thoughts are changing all of the time. I have come to different conclusions.

ADAM: Don't get me wrong, I am happy about it. It was very moving for me when I saw your text. It was just surprising because when we talked about this only 2 weeks ago, your attitude was different. I was wondering what happened that caused the switch?

FATHER: Look, I don't know. I don't understand everything about the process I am going through. It is just how I feel. I don't know how to explain every single thing. I am not just doing it for you. I want to go to that demonstration for myself.

MOTHER (*speaks to therapist*): By the way, I didn't know anything about this. He made that decision and contacted Adam all by himself. It was completely his initiative.

FATHER: I identify with the cause. I guess, somewhere inside, I can imagine that Adam will someday be in that position. I think it is only fair.

THERAPIST (*speaks to Adam*): Can you tell Dad more about how you felt when he sent you that text?

ADAM (*speaks directly to his father*): I was with Oren [his partner] at the time. I told him. I was excited. I am really excited about your wanting to come, but it is also strange. It is important to me because I feel like it is so unjust that the country is telling me that I can't be a father, and I know inside that I will make a great father.

FATHER: That is true. (*Turns to therapist*) Adam would be a great father. He is great with kids, and kids gravitate to him. (*Turns back to Adam*): I have no doubt that you will be a great father.

MOTHER: I completely agree. I am ready for him to be a father tomorrow! Whatever he needs to make it happen, I am right beside him.

In the preceding segment, the father's clear commitment to his son's welfare and his explicit support of Adam's becoming a parent have created a safe enough environment for Adam to then reveal his previously unexpressed fear that his father would abandon him in the future if he got married and had children:

THERAPIST (*speaks to Adam*):   Is that something you are thinking about: having children?

ADAM: Absolutely. Not right now, but it is something I think about for the future. (*Turns to speak directly with his father*) It is also one of my fears about you. With the messages you have given me over the years, I don't really know what to expect when I get to that point. That is definitely one of my big fears.

THERAPIST: What exactly is the fear?

ADAM (*speaks to his father*):   That you will not want to take a part in that.

FATHER: In what?

ADAM: That you will not acknowledge my partner, our relationship, and our kids.

FATHER: In regards to couplehood, I think I have gone through a process and do accept that, even though it seems like you still have doubts about my position on that. In regards to a wedding, I don't know how comfortable I will feel.

THERAPIST: Adam, correct me if I am wrong, but it sounds like you are asking Dad, "If I reach the point that I want to have kids and raise a family, will you be there by my side, a part of that"?

FATHER (*speaks to Adam*):   What do you think the answer to that question is?

ADAM (*speaks to his father*):   I really don't know.

FATHER (*speaks to Adam*):   Then let me make it perfectly clear: I have no doubt that I will be by your side.

ADAM (*eyes tear up*):   That makes me happy to hear. It moves me.

Later in the session:

FATHER (*speaks to Adam*):   I want you to be able to tell me things, even if you are afraid that it will hurt me. You don't need to worry about me anymore. You are a grown man. You can teach me things. In some ways, it is a shame that we needed to come here to reach this point. . . .

ADAM (*smiles*): No, we definitely needed to come here (*laughs*). What I do want to ask from you is that, if I do share things with you . . . not to use those things against me to support your position. For example, if I tell you something is hard, I am afraid that you will tell me, "You see, I told you that you should keep a low profile." I know that it comes from a place of worry, but it constricts me. Sometimes things are hard, but that is my choice, that is what allows me to be me, to grow.

FATHER: Today, I know how to respond better. I will still worry. There is still an urge to protect you. But I know how to stop myself and pick my words. To be there in the way that you need me to. I understand now that not every time you come to share something, you are coming for a solution or for help. Sometimes it is just about sharing. In the past, I think I felt like I had to always give you advice, solve something. Now I know that I just need to stand by your side and be proud. If you need my help, you know how to ask. I always believed in you. I am sure that you will succeed. The problem is me. So, I need to work on myself.

ADAM (*turns to both of his parents*): I love you guys.

THERAPIST: I can see how much love there is between you all. It is really heartwarming. I wanted to go back to what you (*speaks to father*) said a few minutes ago about the wedding and ask you in what ways you think it might be hard for you. I imagine that brings up questions and worries for Adam. That maybe you won't be at the wedding. That it will be too much for you to tolerate. That he can't necessarily count on you definitely being there.

FATHER: I have no doubt that I will be there. Adam is the most important thing in my life, along with my wife and other children. There is nothing that is going to come between us.

ADDRESSING LESS THAN OPTIMAL OUTCOMES

As with any type of therapy, not every case is successful. Far from it. In the open trial of attachment-based family therapy for sexual and gender minority young adults and their nonaccepting parents (G. M. Diamond et al., 2022) described in Chapter 2, the authors found that approximately one quarter of the young adults did not report any improvement in parental acceptance or rejection. Even among those families that benefit, there is range in the magnitude of gains made. Sometime outcomes are modest, circumscribed, and mixed. For example, at the end of therapy, parents may be better able to understand and validate their young adult's frustration and legitimate unmet needs but still feel unable to fully meet those needs. This was the situation with one deeply religious family that participated in the clinical trial. The son, a yeshiva student, conveyed to his mother how important it was for him to know that she accepted that he was gay and know that she would remain positively involved in his life. It was particularly important to him to be able to consult with her about potential romantic partners. This young man had no experience with romantic relationships and, like many in his religious community, looked to his family for support and direction in such matters. He had a deep appreciation of his mother's ability to judge character and felt like he needed her guidance to make sure that he chose a good-hearted, honest man.

Over the course of treatment, his mother was able to hear—for the first time—her son's experience of coming out to himself and the struggles he went through before acknowledging to himself that he was gay and that it was not going to change. As the treatment advanced, she became less overwhelmed, more compassionate, and more committed to supporting her son to the best of her ability. At the same time, she was still unable to reconcile her religious beliefs and her son's sexual orientation, saying, "It just isn't something that is acceptable in our community. It is a sin according to the Bible." She also felt like it quickly became too much for her when her son spoke about his friends from the LGBTQ+ community and his desire to be in a committed romantic relationship with another man.

During the fifth task of treatment, they were able to negotiate boundaries that were satisfactory for both of them and strategize regarding how to approach future sensitive conversations. For example, they agreed that if mother felt like her son was sharing too many personal details about his life as a gay man, and she was getting overwhelmed, she would tell him. They would then pause the conversation until she felt like she could listen again. Mother also told her son that if he referred to potential partners as "friends" rather than as "boyfriends," it would be easier for her to hear what he had to say and provide the consultation he sought. Although this outcome is not ideal, the change felt huge for the family. By the end of treatment, mother felt less distress, and her son felt more secure that his mother would remain by his side and continue to support and guide him as needed.

In some cases, however, parents fail to become more accepting over the course of the treatment, and there is no improvement in the young adult–parent relationship. Parents continue to be dominated by their fear, shame, anger, loss, and sense of hopelessness. They perceive themselves as victims or failures. They feel criticized, disrespected, unappreciated, or attacked. In turn, they become defensive and controlling. They remain more focused on their own despair than on their young adult's experience. Consequently, they are unable to hear and empathically respond to their young adult's pain and unmet needs.

Behaviorally, nothing changes. These parents continue to avoid coming into contact with any aspect of their young adult's life that has to do with their sexual orientation or gender identity. They still refuse to meet or interact with their young adult's partner and are unwilling to hear about their young adult's friends, interests, or activities. They may tenaciously hold on to the belief that their young adult's sexual orientation or gender identity is a choice and that if their young adult had better sense, stronger character, cared enough, or was not so selfish, they would work harder to change it. Others may see it as a biological defect. In any case, they continue to view being gay or genderqueer as abnormal, a liability, and something to be ashamed of. Often, these parents fantasize about having a relationship with their young adult that is separate and disconnected from their young adult's sexual orientation or gender identity.

As a result of their parents' continued rejection, the young adult continues to feel frustrated, unseen, unheard, and rejected, and the rupture in the relationship remains unresolved. In such cases, this last stage of treatment is devoted to meeting alone with the young adult and validating and processing their disappointment, frustration, assertive anger, loss, and grief. In the following segment, a young woman, Shira, talks with the therapist about her parents and her partner, Emma:

THERAPIST: How did you feel after our meeting together with your parents?

SHIRA [daughter]:   It was so frustrating. It is like banging my head against the wall. I'm trying to tell them how screwed up it is that me and Emma are sitting alone in our apartment on holidays and that they are all together having a grand old time.

THERAPIST: I thought you did a really good job of telling your parents how hurt and alone you feel in those moments. You were clear, you did not attack them, and you spoke from your heart. I saw that it was hard for them to listen. That they got into this defensive mode and weren't really able to hear or acknowledge your feelings—that they were more focused on explaining all of the reasons why it was hard for them and why you and Emma couldn't be there. It must have been really frustrating, disappointing.

SHIRA [daughter]:   What the heck! Why did they even bother having kids? What kind of parents cut their children out of the family just so that they can maintain this facade of normalcy, perfection? You have a daughter, and you are more concerned about what other people think? What your brothers who you see twice a year think? They are more important to you than your own daughter?

Having the therapist present to witness their parents' inability to respond empathically can be therapeutic for the young adult. The therapist was there with them and saw and felt the same thing. They can validate the adult child's experience. Suddenly, it is not just in their own minds. It is a shared experience. They do not feel crazy anymore. They did the best they could, and their parents still could not understand or acknowledge their feelings and needs. It is no longer about them finding the "right" approach or perfect way of saying it. They now know that they have given it their best shot. There is something freeing about knowing that you have done all that you can do—everything in your power—even if things did not work out as you had hoped.

Indeed, many of these young adults have spent years trying to figure out how to get through to their parents to no avail. After doing all in their power during the attachment tasks, there is a sense of relief—even if things did not work out how they had hoped. They feel a sense of being able to let go. This process of letting go, however, also elicits deep sadness and grief. The young adult comes face to face with the loss in their relationship with their parents. They have to mourn. For some, it is the loss of what was once a warm, safe, caring, and protective bond. Even for those who were never close with their parents, it is the loss of the dream that their parents might one day fully understand their feelings and needs, put their own fears and shame aside, and be there for and with them in a way that they have not been in the past:

SHIRA [daughter]:   They are going to miss out on being a part of my life. It is *their* loss. I am going to take care of myself. Emma and I are going to move on with our lives. I am not going to let them hold me back.

THERAPIST: Yes. They are going to miss out on having you in their life. I agree that you and Emma need to take care of yourselves and each other and focus on your relationship. She is a real support for you. It is really sad that it all worked out that way. I know how close you used to be with both of your parents.

SHIRA [daughter] (*begins to cry profusely*):   I realize that I can't count on them anymore. I used to feel that, no matter what happened, I had my parents to turn to. Now, that is gone. I don't have that anymore.

THERAPIST: That must really hurt.

This is a hard and painful process both for the adult child and for the therapist. It is heart-wrenching to watch as a young adult comes to the realization that their parents are limited; that their relationship with their parents is conditional; and that their parents are not currently able or willing to provide them with the recognition, empathy, admiration, love, and support that they so desire and deserve. These moments can evoke intense affect. The role of the therapist is to mirror, contain, and validate the young adult's adaptive grief and assertive anger.

Once the young adult has sufficiently processed their adaptive grief and anger, the therapist then helps them plan how to manage any future interactions they might have with their parents. Sometimes this means strategizing about how to protect themselves. In some cases, the young adult will choose to limit contact with one or both of their parents, refrain from talking about certain topics, or make contact conditional on certain basic rules of common decency and mutual respect. The therapist and young adult think together about how the young adult can adjust their expectations and set limits so that they are not disappointed or hurt in the future, while at the same time remaining open for any signals that their parents are ready for change. When indicated, the therapist will also spend time helping the young adult identify new sources of support, including LGBTQ+-affirmative support groups and counseling services.

8 SPECIAL CLINICAL ISSUES

The description of attachment-based family therapy for sexual and gender minority young adults and their nonaccepting parents (ABFT-SGM) and clinical illustrations presented in this book reflect the core elements of the treatment model. However, as with any treatment model, special clinical issues can arise that require therapists' attention, acumen, and flexibility. This chapter touches on a few of these not uncommon clinical circumstances.

MARITAL CONFLICT AND SPLIT LOYALTIES

It is natural, perhaps inevitable, for parents to be in different places on the acceptance continuum, both at the start of treatment and when it ends. Each parent has their own personality, life experience, and belief system. Therefore, they respond differently to their young adult's same-sex orientation or nonconforming gender identity. Ideally, over the course of therapy, both parents make progress toward greater acceptance—in tandem and as a team. Often, a more accepting parent helps their less accepting partner by providing

https://doi.org/10.1037/0000352-008
Attachment-Based Family Therapy for Sexual and Gender Minority Young Adults and Their Nonaccepting Parents, by G. M. Diamond and R. Boruchovitz-Zamir

support, empathy, and reassurance. Other times, the more accepting parent may set limits and takes a stand vis-à-vis their less accepting partner (e.g., "We are having his partner over for the holidays, and there is no other option. I will not have him be alone on New Year's"). More accepting parents can serve as a catalyst by disconfirming their less accepting partner's catastrophic fantasies, soothing their fears, and modeling courage and acceptance. They remind them of the price that their young adult and the family as a whole are paying because of their nonacceptance.

In some families, however, large disparities between parents' levels of acceptance and motivation to change can lead to severe conflict and power struggles. Such was the case in the Malul family, for example, in which the daughter had come out as a lesbian more than 8 years earlier and was currently living with her partner. Over the course of the treatment, the mother was able to connect to, empathize with, and validate her young adult daughter's sense of hurt, anger, loss, grief, and anxiety associated with not feeling accepted. This, in turn, motivated her to be more accepting and supportive of her daughter. Her husband, on the other hand, remained unyielding in his rejection of his daughter's sexual orientation, even after the attachment task. He tenaciously held on to the belief that she was not really a lesbian— that she had chosen the "easy way out" just like everything else she had done in her life. He refused to allow her to bring her partner to their family home, did not want to hear anything about what was going on in her personal life, and refused to provide her with any financial or other support as long as she was living with a woman.

Such dynamics can have a devastating effect on the marital relationship, the young adult, and the integrity of the family as a whole. In the case of the Malul family, the mother was furious at, and disappointed in, her husband. She accused him of abandoning their daughter and putting her at risk just because he could not overcome his own shame and rigid beliefs. The father, for his part, dismissed his wife's concerns, demeaning her for being soft and enabling their daughter. The daughter felt invalidated and coerced by her father and abandoned by her mother. She was disappointed in her mother for not being stronger and standing up to her father. The mother felt torn between her loyalty to her husband, on the one hand, and her loyalty to her daughter, on the other hand. She felt like she was stuck between a rock and hard place with no way out. She felt powerless to get her husband to change and did not want to leave him alone in his distress. At the same time, she wanted to support her daughter in her moment of need. To make matters worse, the father had developed an unholy alliance with his eldest son, whose role it was to support his father's rejecting position and join him in berating his mother and excluding his sister.

In such cases, the ABFT-SGM therapist scales back the treatment goals. We shift from trying to facilitate greater acceptance on the part of the rejecting parent to trying to help parents extricate themselves from the deadlock they have found themselves in. The goal becomes to find a new status quo that is at least tolerable for all family members. To unbalance the system and create urgency, we meet with parents alone without the young adult present and reflect to them the enormous price that they and their young adult are paying because of their ongoing conflicts and power struggles.

In the example with the Malul family, the therapist empathically reflected the father's feelings of helplessness but, at the same time, challenged his behaviors—the way he was responding. The therapist predicted that if he remained intransigent and controlling, it would only lead to greater misery and, potentially, the dissolution of the marriage, a complete cutoff from his daughter, or some other tragedy.

This type of intervention usually resonates because it is real and true. It accurately captures and heightens the two sides of the rejecting parent's dilemma, of their internal conflict. Typically, such interventions evoke in the nonaccepting parent a desire to find some type of compromise solution—some way to protect themselves from feeling ashamed or out of control while at the same time meeting some of their partner's and young adult's needs.

In the Malul family, for example, the father ended up agreeing that his wife would give their daughter a certain amount of money until she found a better-paying job. Also, even though the father continued to express his disapproval of his daughter's relationship with her partner, he agreed that the two of them could come to their home for the holidays. The mother, on her part, decided that she would start meeting regularly with her daughter alone at her daughter's apartment.

Although far from perfect, this compromise led to a reduction in marital conflict, allowed the mother to provide more support to her daughter, and left her daughter feeling more connected and taken care of. Moreover, the mother's increased acceptance and assertive stance vis-à-vis her husband changed the very way her daughter perceived her. By the end of the treatment, the daughter viewed her mother as stronger, more committed to supporting her, and able to protect her in ways she had not in the past. Her mother felt freer to support her daughter without feeling like she was endangering the integrity of the family as a whole.

SIBLINGS

Many times, ABFT-SGM therapists are asked if we include the young adult's siblings in the treatment. The answer is, "Not typically, but sometimes—when it is indicated." The core focus of ABFT-SGM is on promoting parental acceptance and transforming relationships between the young adult and their parents. Therefore, the work centers on helping the young adult share their experience of not feeling accepted or connected and on helping parents listen, understand, empathize, and respond in a validating manner. For that reason, siblings are typically not involved in the treatment.

However, in certain circumstances, the young adult, together with the therapist, may decide to invite one or more of the young adult's siblings to come in for a session or two during the later stages of the therapy. In some cases, this is because the friction between the young adult and their sibling is a major stressor in the young adult's life and contributes to their feeling unaccepted and disconnected from the family. This was the case with Ben, a 35-year-old gay man and his younger brother.

Ben reported that he and his brother had been close growing up. However, since he had come out 2 years before, his brother had become increasingly distant from him. When they did have contact at family events or during weekend dinners at their parents' home, his brother was nasty toward him, making sarcastic homophobic comments. Ben was both angry at and hurt by his brother's behavior. He was also sad about the loss of what was once a meaningful bond.

In an effort to work through and resolve this sibling conflict, Ben and his therapist decided to invite his brother to a session—just the two of them. During the session, Ben was able to effectively convey his feelings of hurt, legitimate anger, and loss directly to his brother. His brother, after initially being defensive, was gradually able to hear and validate some of Ben's feelings. The therapist also explored with Ben's brother what it had been like for him when Ben came out. His brother was able to say that he was surprised, taken aback, and confused by Ben's coming out. He did not really know how to react. He acknowledged also feeling a sense of loss but was ambivalent about whether he wanted to get close to Ben again. By the end of the session, Ben's brother had a better sense of how his behavior had affected Ben over the years. He was empathic and showed remorse and also expressed a commitment to at least being more civil and respectful to Ben.

In other instances, the therapist raises the possibility of inviting one or more of the young adult's siblings to a session because we think that they can be important allies. Siblings can be a unique source of support. They often know the young adult better than anybody else and have shared the experience of growing up under the same roof with the same parents. They have witnessed the interactions between their brother or sister and their parents. Therefore, they can understand, identify with, and validate the young adults' frustration, hurt, and longing in a way that most others cannot. They also often have useful insights regarding their parents' personalities, how to approach their parents in a productive manner, and the issues that need to be talked about. Because they are part of the family system, they are in the position to intervene, mediate, and advocate for the young adult, when appropriate.

MENTAL HEALTH

In many families, one or both parents suffer from significant mental health challenges, including depression, anxiety, posttraumatic stress disorder, and personality disorders. Even when parents do not meet formal diagnostic criteria, they may have high levels of anxiety symptoms; be extremely avoidant, dependent, or rigid; or quickly decompensate in stressful, highly arousing situations. Mental health challenges can impede parents' ability to productively participate in the therapy process. It can make it hard for them to stay focused; reflect on their child's state of mind; differentiate between their own needs and those of their young adult; be empathic; validate their young adult's experience; and take responsibility for their own rejecting, nonattuned responses. These parents easily feel criticized, attacked, or misunderstood. They may quickly become overwhelmed or defensive, blaming and attacking.

The therapist needs to work especially hard to support, soothe, and redirect such parents on a moment-by-moment basis. We also need to set the treatment goals according to parents' psychological and emotional capacities. In some cases, this may mean less of a focus on experiential work and more parent psychoeducation. When indicated, we also help these parents access appropriate adjunct clinical services and support in the community. In some instances, we refer them to individual therapy. In other instances, we refer them to lesbian, gay, bisexual, transgender, and queer (LGBTQ+)–affirmative parent support groups, such as PFLAG. Throughout our work with such parents, we maintain a nonjudgmental posture and keep in mind that what might seem like only small changes in their ability to hear and validate their young adult's experience can mean the world to their young adult.

In other cases, it is the young adults themselves who are struggling with mental health issues. This is not uncommon. As mentioned earlier in

Chapter 1, an abundance of research over the past 2 decades has shown the robust link between identifying as LGBTQ+ and psychological symptoms, including depression, anxiety, rejection sensitivity, and suicidal ideation. This link is commonly attributed to minority stress. Indeed, some of the young adults presenting for ABFT-SGM have suffered from years of victimization and trauma. They have been ridiculed, emotionally abused, threatened, and physically assaulted at school, in public spaces, and even within their own families. They have been, and still are, subjected to discrimination, prejudice, and homo[trans]phobia. Consequently, they may be hypervigilant, suspicious, agitated, dysregulated, and quick to lash out. They may find it hard to trust others, including their parents. They may be extremely sensitive to criticism and reactive to any hint of empathic failure.

In such cases, it is the therapist's job to normalize the young adult's experience in light of the severe stressors they have faced and are still facing in their lives. The therapist also works to contain, soothe, and support the young adult so that they can effectively express their feelings and unmet needs and so that they can remain open to hearing their parents' new, more empathic responses. The therapist often spends extra time during individual alliance building sessions with these young adults to teach them emotional regulation strategies, help them to formulate exactly what they want to say to their parents, and prepare them so that they can respond effectively to suboptimal responses from parents. Again, depending on the young adult's level of functioning, the therapist will adjust the pace and intensity of the treatment process and adapt the treatment goals. In such cases, the therapist will be careful to conduct conjoint attachment episodes in a more structured manner, careful to monitor and shape interactions on a moment-by-moment basis.

THE ROLE OF RELIGION

For many parents, reconciling their religious beliefs with their young adult's sexual orientation or gender identity is a major challenge. Indeed, research findings consistently show that higher levels of parents' religiosity are correlated with lower levels of acceptance (Rosenkrantz et al., 2020; Ryan et al., 2010). This may be particularly true for parents of gay men because there are explicit references to male homosexuality being forbidden in the Bible. Such parents face the task of making sense of how God, on the one hand, prohibits certain same-sex acts while, on the other hand, created their son gay or allowed him to be gay.

In work done by ABFT-SGM therapists, we have found that parents who succeed in at least partially resolving the conflict between their religious beliefs and their child's sexual or gender identity often adopt the position that there are simply things that they may never understand. They find comfort in knowing that God has a plan, and they submit to his wisdom and will. Our clinical observations echo findings from studies with conservative Christian parents. For example, Cavallo and Bradley (2018) found that acceptance among such parents was associated with giving over control to God and trusting in the Holy Spirit. In our conversations with religious parents, we help them focus on those core religious values that promote acceptance and connection. For example, Jewish tradition and spiritual writings emphasize the importance of loving others unconditionally, family cohesiveness, living one's truth openly rather than lying or engaging in concealment, and *tikkun olam*: working toward making the world kinder and more just. Likewise, Cavallo and Bradley found that among conservative Christian parents, acceptance was based on values, such as loving a person as they are, not as we would have them be, and on not being judgmental. Jewish tradition also espouses that it is not good for a person to be on their own alone in the world—that everybody should have a partner. Highlighting this particular core value is especially helpful for parents who have a hard time accepting their young adult's same-sex romantic partner.

Parents who live in conservative, tight-knit, religious communities not only have to resolve their internal conflict between their religious beliefs and their young adult's identity, but also have to cope with the negative responses from others around them. These can include judgmental, homo[trans]phobic, intolerant attitudes and comments by neighbors, friends, and even religious leaders. Some parents may also face social rejection. Their family may no longer be invited to certain friends' homes for dinner. Their other children's opportunities for dating and marriage may be diminished. Needless to say, this can exacerbate parents' experience of shame and fear and make it harder for them to be more open and accepting.

Yet another challenge for religious parents is that their LGBTQ+ young adults often become less religious over time. Some continue to practice their religion but join less orthodox or less traditional churches or synagogues. Others become altogether secular and leave their religious upbringing behind. For religious parents, this feels like a double loss. Not only have they lost their hetero(cisgender)-normative dream of having their young adult marry an opposite-sex spouse and bring biological children (grandchildren) into the family fold, but they also feel like they have lost the connection to their young adult that was based on shared religious values and traditions. A cultural chasm forms. This makes it even harder for parents to understand and accept their lesbian, gay, bisexual, transgender, or queer young adult and maintain a close relationship with them. In almost every religious family that we have worked with, parents reported that their young adult's becoming less religious felt like a greater loss and was more difficult to cope with than their young adult's minority sexual or gender identity. With such families, we search for common values that still bond the young adult and their parents, such as the importance of family, spending time together, a sense of belonging, and mutual respect and support.

FLUID, NONEXCLUSIVE, AND NONBINARY IDENTITIES

In our (GMD, RBZ, and our colleagues') clinical work, we have found that parents have a more difficult time accepting their young adult's identity when it does not easily fit into parents' preconceived notions of sexual orientation and gender. More specifically, we have found that parents have a harder time accepting bisexual and genderqueer young adults and young adults who choose not to define themselves than those who identify as gay or lesbian. We have heard more than one father say,

> If she were to just tell me definitively that she was lesbian, I would accept it and move on. But she doesn't say that. She keeps saying that, right now, she is in love with a woman but that she doesn't want to define herself. That she is attracted to people, regardless of their gender. She is obviously still confused, still unsure herself. The last thing that I want to do is show my acceptance. That will only give her permission and push her in the wrong direction.

Other parents have said things like the following:

> She defines herself as bisexual. She has had boyfriends, serious relationships with men in the past. We know that right now she is with a woman, but we still hope that will change, and she will end up being with a man.

Indeed, findings from a study Samarova et al. (2014) conducted on Israeli young adults revealed that although parents' acceptance of their gay and lesbian young adults improved over time, the same was not true for parents of bisexual young adults.

Our clinical experience is that parents have a hard time accepting their young adults' nonbinary, nonexclusive, and fluid sexual orientations and gender identities for at least two reasons. First, such identities seemingly leave open the possibility that things might shift or change in the future.

There is no finality for parents, no resolution. This makes it harder for some parents to come to terms with their loss, mourn, cope, and move on. They get stuck holding onto hope that their young adult will eventually adopt a heteronormative, gender conforming identity and lifestyle and that their own life will return to "normal." Second, and relatedly, many parents have a hard time imagining, understanding, and connecting to the experience of being attracted to a range of genders or being gender fluid. For parents who are exclusively heterosexual and cisgender and who grew up in a world in which sexual attraction and gender identity were rarely explored openly, such experiences of self feel abstract, academic, and almost unreal.

In our work with such families, we try to help the young adult convey their experience of gender and sexuality—what it feels like for them to be nonbinary, bisexual, or queer in some sense of the word; how it is manifested in their daily life; how it is part of their being, of who they are. At the same time, we help parents be curious and listen openly. When therapy goes well, parents rediscover their young adult and the relationship becomes more real. Likewise, young adults finally feel fully seen, appreciated, safe, loved, and admired for who they are.

CONCLUDING THOUGHTS

Deep down, everyone wants to feel seen, loved, and admired by their parents. We want our parents to not only accept us but to be proud of us, revel in who we are as people. We want to know that they are interested in what is going on in our lives and that they feel joy when we are happy and pain when we are hurting. We want to know that they will be there to celebrate with us in good times and support us in bad times. The need to feel seen, recognized, and admired and the need to feel connected, belonging, supported, and safe in the world are fundamental human needs. Parents are our first and most important source for getting those needs met. From the moment we are born, they are our mirrors. They signal to us that we are safe to explore and be our authentic selves and that we are valuable and special just the way we are. Our need for their esteem and to feel connected to them is primal and deep rooted. Even after we become adults and have formed new attachments with romantic partners, friends, colleagues, and mentors, our longing for our parents' emotional investment in us, recognition, unconditional love, support, and admiration is unrivaled. It never wanes.

For LGBTQ+ individuals, being seen, loved, prized by, and connected to their parents may be especially important. Our society is replete with heterosexist and homo[trans]phobic messages that are then internalized and can diminish one's sense of self. When people also feel diminished or outright rejected by their own parents, it is devastating. In contrast, parental acceptance, affirmation, admiration, support, and protection provide a secure base. It is a like having a superpower one can carry around to combat and mitigate homophobia and transphobia, prejudice, discrimination, and hate. Parental acceptance and support not only buffers against the effects of such minority stress, but provides an environment in which the young adult feels safe enough to explore their identity, be vulnerable, form intimate relationships, express their emotions and needs, and connect with others in a meaningful, open, authentic manner.

ABFT-SGM was designed to help parents work through their fear, shame, and helplessness so that they can help their lesbian, gay, bisexual, transgender, or queer young adult feel safe, connected, and prized for who they are. Although not every family finds the therapy helpful, the effort is worth it. Relationships with parents are just too important to give up on without trying. When the process goes well, as it often does, parents end up feeling relief and joy that they have their child back and their family is whole again. Young adults end up feeling understood, respected, loved, and reconnected to their family. They feel liberated, free to be who they want to be. Indeed, at the end of therapy, families frequently tell their therapists that they feel like the work saved their life and their family. In those moments, we are honored, deeply moved, grateful, and humbly reminded of the Talmudic teaching: "He who saves a single life, saves the world entire" (Guggenheimer, 2000).

References

Aquilino, W. S. (2006). Family relationships and support systems in emerging adulthood. In J. J. Arnett & J. L. Tanner (Eds.), *Emerging adults in America: Coming of age in the 21st century* (pp. 193–217). American Psychological Association. https://doi.org/10.1037/11381-008

Arnett, J. J. (2000). Emerging adulthood: A theory of development from the late teens through the twenties. *American Psychologist, 55*(5), 469–480. https://doi.org/10.1037/0003-066X.55.5.469

Arnett, J. J. (2014). *Emerging adulthood: The winding road from the late teens through the twenties.* Oxford University Press. https://doi.org/10.1093/acprof:oso/9780199929382.001.0001

Arnett, J. J., & Schwab, J. (2012). *The Clark University poll of emerging adults: Thriving, struggling, and hopeful.* Clark University.

Balsam, K. F., Molina, Y., Beadnell, B., Simoni, J., & Walters, K. (2011). Measuring multiple minority stress: The LGBT People of Color Microaggressions Scale. *Cultural Diversity & Ethnic Minority Psychology, 17*(2), 163–174. https://doi.org/10.1037/a0023244

Beals, K. P., & Peplau, L. A. (2006). Disclosure patterns within social networks of gay men and lesbians. *Journal of Homosexuality, 51*(2), 101–120. https://doi.org/10.1300/J082v51n02_06

Beck, A. T., Ward, C., Mendleson, M., Mock, J., & Erbaugh, J. (1961). An inventory for measuring depression (BDI). *Archives of General Psychiatry, 4*(6), 561–571. https://doi.org/10.1001/archpsyc.1961.01710120031004

Bordin, E. S. (1994). Theory and research on the therapeutic working alliance: New directions. In A. O. Horvath & L. S. Greenberg (Eds.), *The working alliance: Theory, research, and practice* (pp. 13–37). John Wiley & Sons.

Boruchovitz-Zamir, R., & Diamond, G. M. (2019, September 19–21). *Relationship-focused therapy for sexual minority individuals and their non-accepting parents: Changes in parental positive and negative responses over time* [Paper presentation]. Society for Psychotherapy Research 5th Joint European & UK Chapters Conference, Krakow, Poland.

Bouris, A., Guilamo-Ramos, V., Pickard, A., Shiu, C., Loosier, P. S., Dittus, P., Gloppen, K., & Waldmiller, J. M. (2010). A systematic review of parental influences on the health and well-being of lesbian, gay, and bisexual youth: Time for a new public health research and practice agenda. *The Journal of Primary Prevention, 31*(5–6), 273–309. https://doi.org/10.1007/s10935-010-0229-1

Bowlby, J. (1988). *A secure base: Parent–child attachment and healthy human development*. Basic Books.

Brent, D. A., & Kolko, D. J. (1991). *Supportive relationship treatment manual* [Unpublished manual]. Department of Psychiatry, University of Pittsburgh/ Western Psychiatric Institute and Clinic.

Cavallo, F. J., & Bradley, C. (2018). Examining the therapeutic processes associated with conservative Christian parental acceptance of their son or daughter's lesbian, gay, or bisexual orientation. *The Family Journal, 26*(3), 315–323. https://doi.org/10.1177/1066480718785914

Clark, K. A., Dougherty, L. R., & Pachankis, J. E. (2021). A study of parents of sexual and gender minority children: Linking parental reactions with child mental health. *Psychology of Sexual Orientation and Gender Diversity*. Advance online publication. https://doi.org/10.1037/sgd0000456

Cramer, D. W., & Roach, A. J. (1988). Coming out to mom and dad: A study of gay males and their relationships with their parents. *Journal of Homosexuality, 15*(3–4), 79–92. https://doi.org/10.1300/J082v15n03_04

Crenshaw, K. (1991). Mapping the margins: Identity politics, intersectionality, and violence against women. *Stanford Law Review, 43*(6), 1241–1299. https://doi.org/10.2307/1229039

D'Amico, E., & Julien, D. (2012). Disclosure of sexual orientation and gay, lesbian, and bisexual youths' adjustment: Associations with past and current parental acceptance and rejection. *Journal of GLBT Family Studies, 8*(3), 215–242. https://doi.org/10.1080/1550428X.2012.677232

D'Augelli, A. R. (2002). Mental health problems among lesbian, gay, and bisexual youths ages 14 to 21. *Clinical Child Psychology and Psychiatry, 7*(3), 433–456. https://doi.org/10.1177/1359104502007003039

D'Augelli, A. R., Grossman, A. H., Salter, N. P., Vasey, J. J., Starks, M. T., & Sinclair, K. O. (2005). Predicting the suicide attempts of lesbian, gay, and bisexual youth. *Suicide & Life-Threatening Behavior, 35*(6), 646–660. https://doi.org/10.1521/suli.2005.35.6.646

Davis, S. D., & Butler, M. H. (2004). Enacting relationships in marriage and family therapy: A conceptual and operational definition of an enactment. *Journal of Marital and Family Therapy, 30*(3), 319–333. https://doi.org/10.1111/j.1752-0606.2004.tb01243.x

Diamond, G., Creed, T., Gillham, J., Gallop, R., & Hamilton, J. L. (2012). Sexual trauma history does not moderate treatment outcome in attachment-based family therapy (ABFT) for adolescents with suicide ideation. *Journal of Family Psychology, 26*(4), 595–605. https://doi.org/10.1037/a0028414

Diamond, G., Diamond, G. M., & Levy, S. (2021). Attachment-based family therapy: Theory, clinical model, outcomes, and process research. *Journal of Affective Disorders, 294,* 286–295. https://doi.org/10.1016/j.jad.2021.07.005

Diamond, G., & Liddle, H. A. (1996). Resolving a therapeutic impasse between parents and adolescents in multidimensional family therapy. *Journal of Consulting and Clinical Psychology, 64*(3), 481–488. https://doi.org/10.1037/0022-006X.64.3.481

Diamond, G., Siqueland, L., & Diamond, G. M. (2003). Attachment-based family therapy for depressed adolescents: Programmatic treatment development. *Clinical Child and Family Psychology Review, 6*(2), 107–127. https://doi.org/10.1023/A:1023782510786

Diamond, G. M., Boruchovitz-Zamir, R., Gat, I., & Nir-Gottlieb, O. (2019). Relationship-focused therapy for sexual and gender minority individuals and their parents. In J. E. Pachankis & S. A. Safren (Eds.), *Handbook of evidence-based mental health practice with sexual and gender minorities* (pp. 430–456). Oxford University Press.

Diamond, G. M., Boruchovitz-Zamir, R., Nir-Gottlieb, O., Gat, I., Bar-Kalifa, E., Fitoussi, P.-Y., & Katz, S. (2022). Attachment-based family therapy for sexual and gender minority young adults and their nonaccepting parents. *Family Process, 61*(2), 530–548. https://doi.org/10.1111/famp.12770

Diamond, G. M., Diamond, G. S., Levy, S., Closs, C., Ladipo, T., & Siqueland, L. (2012). Attachment-based family therapy for suicidal lesbian, gay, and bisexual adolescents: A treatment development study and open trial with preliminary findings. *Psychotherapy, 49*(1), 62–71. https://doi.org/10.1037/a0026247

Diamond, G. M., Shahar, B., Sabo, D., & Tsvieli, N. (2016). Attachment-based family therapy and emotion-focused therapy for unresolved anger: The role of productive emotional processing. *Psychotherapy, 53*(1), 34–44. https://doi.org/10.1037/pst0000025

Diamond, G. S., Diamond, G. M., & Levy, S. A. (2014). *Attachment-based family therapy for depressed adolescents.* American Psychological Association. https://doi.org/10.1037/14296-000

Diamond, G. S., Kobak, R. R., Krauthamer Ewing, E. S., Levy, S. A., Herres, J. L., Russon, J. M., & Gallop, R. J. (2019). A randomized controlled trial: Attachment-based family and nondirective supportive treatments for youth who are suicidal. *Journal of the American Academy of Child & Adolescent Psychiatry, 58*(7), 721–731. https://doi.org/10.1016/j.jaac.2018.10.006

Diamond, G. S., Reis, B. F., Diamond, G. M., Siqueland, L., & Isaacs, L. (2002). Attachment-based family therapy for depressed adolescents: A treatment development study. *Journal of the American Academy of Child & Adolescent Psychiatry, 41*(10), 1190–1196. https://doi.org/10.1097/00004583-200210000-00008

Diamond, G. S., & Stern, R. S. (2003). Attachment-based family therapy for depressed adolescents: Repairing attachment failures. In S. M. Johnson & V. E. Whiffen (Eds.), *Attachment processes in couple and family therapy* (pp. 191–212). Guilford Press.

Diamond, G. S., Wintersteen, M. B., Brown, G. K., Diamond, G. M., Gallop, R., Shelef, K., & Levy, S. (2010). Attachment-based family therapy for adolescents with suicidal ideation: A randomized controlled trial. *Journal of the American Academy of Child & Adolescent Psychiatry, 49*(2), 122–131. https://doi.org/10.1016/j.jaac.2009.11.002

Diamond, L. M. (2006). What we got wrong about sexual identity development: Unexpected findings from a longitudinal study of young women. In A. M. Omoto & H. S. Kurtzman (Eds.), *Sexual orientation and mental health: Examining identity and development in lesbian, gay and bisexual people* (pp. 73–94). American Psychological Association. https://doi.org/10.1037/11261-004

Diamond, L. M., & Alley, J. (2022). Rethinking minority stress: A social safety perspective on the health effects of stigma in sexually-diverse and gender-diverse populations. *Neuroscience and Biobehavioral Reviews, 138*, 104720. https://doi.org/10.1016/j.neubiorev.2022.104720

Doherty, N. A., & Feeney, J. A. (2004). The composition of attachment networks throughout the adult years. *Personal Relationships, 11*(4), 469–488. https://doi.org/10.1111/j.1475-6811.2004.00093.x

Drumheller, K., & McQuay, B. (2010). Living in the buckle: Promoting LGBT outreach services in conservative urban/rural centers. *Communication Studies, 61*(1), 70–86. https://doi.org/10.1080/10510970903398010

Dvir, N. (2021, February 23). *2020 sees uptick in anti-LGBTQ hate crime.* Israel Hayom. https://www.israelhayom.com/2021/02/23/2020-sees-uptick-in-anti-lgbtq-incidents/

Eisenberg, M. E., & Resnick, M. D. (2006). Suicidality among gay, lesbian and bisexual youth: The role of protective factors. *The Journal of Adolescent Health, 39*(5), 662–668. https://doi.org/10.1016/j.jadohealth.2006.04.024

Eliason, M. J. (2014). An exploration of terminology related to sexuality and gender: Arguments for standardizing the language. *Social Work in Public Health, 29*(2), 162–175. https://doi.org/10.1080/19371918.2013.775887

Elizur, Y., & Ziv, M. (2001). Family support and acceptance, gay male identity formation, and psychological adjustment: A path model. *Family Process, 40*(2), 125–144. https://doi.org/10.1111/j.1545-5300.2001.4020100125.x

Evans, E., Hawton, K., & Rodham, K. (2004). Factors associated with suicidal phenomena in adolescents: A systematic review of population-based studies. *Clinical Psychology Review, 24*(8), 957–979. https://doi.org/10.1016/j.cpr.2004.04.005

Feder, M. M., & Diamond, G. M. (2016). Parent–therapist alliance and parent attachment-promoting behaviour in attachment-based family therapy for suicidal and depressed adolescents. *Journal of Family Therapy, 38*(1), 82–101. https://doi.org/10.1111/1467-6427.12078

Fingerman, K. L., Cheng, Y.-P., Tighe, L., Birditt, K. S., & Zarit, S. (2012). Relationships between young adults and their parents. In A. Booth, S. Brown, N. Landale, W. Manning, & S. McHale (Eds.), *Early adulthood in a family context* (Vol. 2, pp. 59–85). Springer.

Floyd, F. J., Stein, T. S., Harter, K. S. M., Allison, A., & Nye, C. L. (1999). Gay, lesbian, and bisexual youths: Separation-individuation, parental attitudes, identity consolidation, and well-being. *Journal of Youth and Adolescence, 28*(6), 719–739. https://doi.org/10.1023/A:1021691601737

Flückiger, C., Del Re, A. C., Wampold, B. E., & Horvath, A. O. (2018). The alliance in adult psychotherapy: A meta-analytic synthesis. *Psychotherapy, 55*(4), 316–340. https://doi.org/10.1037/pst0000172

Fonagy, P., Steele, H., & Steele, M. (1991). Maternal representations of attachment during pregnancy predict the organization of infant–mother attachment at one year of age. *Child Development, 62*(5), 891–905. https://doi.org/10.2307/1131141

Fonagy, P., Target, M., Steele, H., & Steele, M. (1998). *Reflective-functioning manual, version 5.0, for application to adult attachment interviews.* University College London.

Friedlander, M. L., Escudero, V., Heatherington, L., & Diamond, G. M. (2011). Alliance in couple and family therapy. *Psychotherapy, 48*(1), 25–33. https://doi.org/10.1037/a0022060

Friedlander, M. L., Escudero, V., Horvath, A. O., Heatherington, L., Cabero, A., & Martens, M. P. (2006). System for observing family therapy alliances: A tool for research and practice. *Journal of Counseling Psychology, 53*(2), 214–225. https://doi.org/10.1037/0022-0167.53.2.214

Friedlander, M. L., Escudero, V., Welmers-van de Poll, M. J., & Heatherington, L. (2018). Meta-analysis of the alliance-outcome relation in couple and family therapy. *Psychotherapy, 55*(4), 356–371. https://doi.org/10.1037/pst0000161

Friedlander, M. L., Heatherington, L., & Diamond, G. M. (2021). Systemic and conjoint couple and family therapies: Recent advances and future promise. In M. Barkham, W. Lutz, & L. G. Castonguay (Eds.), *Bergin and Garfield's handbook of psychotherapy and behavior change* (7th ed., pp. 539–581). John Wiley & Sons.

Friedlander, M. L., Heatherington, L., Johnson, B., & Skowron, E. A. (1994). Sustaining engagement: A change event in family therapy. *Journal of Counseling Psychology, 41*(4), 438–448. https://doi.org/10.1037/0022-0167.41.4.438

Gardner, B. C., & Butler, M. H. (2009). Enacting relationships in MFT: The empirical, theoretical, and clinical case for incorporating enactments as common factors in the best practice model. *Journal of Couple & Relationship Therapy, 8*(4), 306–324. https://doi.org/10.1080/15332690903246093

Gottman, J. M., Katz, L. F., & Hooven, C. (1996). Parental meta-emotion philosophy and the emotional life of families: Theoretical models and preliminary data. *Journal of Family Psychology, 10*(3), 243–268. https://doi.org/10.1037/0893-3200.10.3.243

Greenberg, L. S. (2011). *Emotion-focused therapy.* American Psychological Association.

Greenberg, L. S. (2012). Emotions, the great captains of our lives: Their role in the process of change in psychotherapy. *American Psychologist, 67*(8), 697–707. https://doi.org/10.1037/a0029858

Greenberg, L. S. (2017). Emotion-focused therapy of depression. *Person-Centered and Experiential Psychotherapies, 16*(2), 106–117. https://doi.org/10.1080/14779757.2017.1330702

Greenberg, L. S., & Iwakabe, S. (2011). Emotion-focused therapy and shame. In R. L. Dearing & J. P. Tangney (Eds.), *Shame in the therapy hour* (pp. 69–90). American Psychological Association. https://doi.org/10.1037/12326-003

Greenberg, L. S., & Pascual-Leone, A. (2006). Emotion in psychotherapy: A practice-friendly research review. *Journal of Clinical Psychology, 62*(5), 611–630. https://doi.org/10.1002/jclp.20252

Grossman, A. H., Park, J. Y., Frank, J. A., & Russell, S. T. (2021). Parental responses to transgender and gender nonconforming youth: Associations with parent support, parental abuse, and youths' psychological adjustment. *Journal of Homosexuality, 68*(8), 1260–1277. https://doi.org/10.1080/00918369.2019.1696103

Guggenheimer, H. W. (Ed.). (2000). *The Jerusalem Talmud: Edition, translation, and commentary*. Walter de Gruyter.

Hall, W. J. (2018). Psychosocial risk and protective factors for depression among lesbian, gay, bisexual, and queer youth: A systematic review. *Journal of Homosexuality, 65*(3), 263–316. https://doi.org/10.1080/00918369.2017.1317467

Harris, M. A., & Orth, U. (2020). The link between self-esteem and social relationships: A meta-analysis of longitudinal studies. *Journal of Personality and Social Psychology, 119*(6), 1459–1477. https://doi.org/10.1037/pspp0000265

Harvey, R. G., & Stone Fish, L. (2015). Queer youth in family therapy. *Family Process, 54*(3), 396–417. https://doi.org/10.1111/famp.12170

Hatzenbuehler, M. L., Dovidio, J. F., Nolen-Hoeksema, S., & Phills, C. E. (2009). An implicit measure of anti-gay attitudes: Prospective associations with emotion regulation strategies and psychological distress. *Journal of Experimental Social Psychology, 45*(6), 1316–1320. https://doi.org/10.1016/j.jesp.2009.08.005

Heatherington, L., Friedlander, M. L., Diamond, G. M., Escudero, V., & Pinsof, W. M. (2015). 25 years of systemic therapies research: Progress and promise. *Psychotherapy Research, 25*(3), 348–364. https://doi.org/10.1080/10503307.2014.983208

Hershberger, S. L., & D'Augelli, A. R. (1995). The impact of victimization on the mental health and suicidality of lesbian, gay, and bisexual youths. *Developmental Psychology, 31*(1), 65–74. https://doi.org/10.1037/0012-1649.31.1.65

Ibrahim, M., Russon, J., Levy, S., & Diamond, G. (2018). Promoting parental acceptance of bisexuality: A case study of attachment-based family therapy. *Journal of Family Psychotherapy, 29*(3), 223–251. https://doi.org/10.1080/08975353.2018.1427401

Kibrik, E. L., Cohen, N., Stolowicz-Melman, D., Levy, A., Boruchovitz-Zamir, R., & Diamond, G. M. (2019). Measuring adult children's perceptions of their parents' acceptance and rejection of their sexual orientation: Initial development of the Parental Acceptance and Rejection of Sexual Orientation Scale (PARSOS). *Journal of Homosexuality, 66*(11), 1513–1534. https://doi.org/10.1080/00918369.2018.1503460

Kiekens, W., la Roi, C., Bos, H. M. W., Kretschmer, T., van Bergen, D. D., & Veenstra, R. (2020). Explaining health disparities between heterosexual and LGB adolescents by integrating the minority stress and psychological mediation frameworks: Findings from the TRAILS study. *Journal of Youth and Adolescence, 49*(9), 1767–1782. https://doi.org/10.1007/s10964-020-01206-0

Kobak, R., & Bosmans, G. (2019). Attachment and psychopathology: A dynamic model of the insecure cycle. *Current Opinion in Psychology, 25*, 76–80. https://doi.org/10.1016/j.copsyc.2018.02.018

Koepke, S., & Denissen, J. J. (2012). Dynamics of identity development and separation–individuation in parent–child relationships during adolescence and emerging adulthood–A conceptual integration. *Developmental Review, 32*(1), 67–88. https://doi.org/10.1016/j.dr.2012.01.001

Kramer, U., Pascual-Leone, A., Despland, J.-N., & de Roten, Y. (2015). One minute of grief: Emotional processing in short-term dynamic psychotherapy for adjustment disorder. *Journal of Consulting and Clinical Psychology, 83*(1), 187–198. https://doi.org/10.1037/a0037979

LaSala, M. C. (2010). *Coming out, coming home: Helping families adjust to a gay or lesbian child.* Columbia University Press.

Levy, S. A., Russon, J., & Diamond, G. M. (2016). Attachment-based family therapy for suicidal lesbian, gay, and bisexual adolescents: A case study. *Australian & New Zealand Journal of Family Therapy, 37*(2), 190–206. https://doi.org/10.1002/anzf.1151

Liddle, H. A. (2009). Multidimensional family therapy: A science-based treatment system for adolescent drug abuse. In J. H. Bray & M. Stanton (Eds.), *The Wiley-Blackwell handbook of family psychology* (pp. 341–354). Wiley Blackwell. https://psycnet.apa.org/doi/10.1002/9781444310238.ch23

Lifshitz, C., Tsvieli, N., Bar-Kalifa, E., Abbott, C., Diamond, G. S., Kobak, R. R., & Diamond, G. M. (2021). Emotional processing in attachment-based family therapy for suicidal adolescents. *Psychotherapy Research, 31*(2), 267–279. https://doi.org/10.1080/10503307.2020.1745315

Livingston, J., & Fourie, E. (2016). The experiences and meanings that shape heterosexual fathers' relationships with their gay sons in South Africa. *Journal of Homosexuality, 63*(12), 1630–1659. https://doi.org/10.1080/00918369.2016.1158009

Luyckx, K., Soenens, B., Vansteenkiste, M., Goossens, L., & Berzonsky, M. D. (2007). Parental psychological control and dimensions of identity formation in emerging adulthood. *Journal of Family Psychology, 21*(3), 546–550. https://doi.org/10.1037/0893-3200.21.3.546

Luyten, P., Mayes, L. C., Nijssens, L., & Fonagy, P. (2017). The parental reflective functioning questionnaire: Development and preliminary validation. *PLOS ONE*, *12*(5), Article e0176218. https://doi.org/10.1371/journal.pone.0176218

McConnell, E. A., Janulis, P., Phillips, G., II, Truong, R., & Birkett, M. (2018). Multiple minority stress and LGBT community resilience among sexual minority men. *Psychology of Sexual Orientation and Gender Diversity*, *5*(1), 1–12. https://doi.org/10.1037/sgd0000265

McKinnon, J. M., & Greenberg, L. S. (2017). Vulnerable emotional expression in emotion focused couples therapy: Relating interactional processes to outcome. *Journal of Marital and Family Therapy*, *43*(2), 198–212. https://doi.org/10.1111/jmft.12229

Meneses, C. W., & Greenberg, L. S. (2011). The construction of a model of the process of couples' forgiveness in emotion-focused therapy for couples. *Journal of Marital and Family Therapy*, *37*(4), 491–502. https://doi.org/10.1111/j.1752-0606.2011.00234.x

Meyer, I. H. (2003). Prejudice, social stress, and mental health in lesbian, gay, and bisexual populations: Conceptual issues and research evidence. *Psychological Bulletin*, *129*(5), 674–697. https://doi.org/10.1037/0033-2909.129.5.674

Minuchin, S. (1974). *Families & family therapy*. Harvard University Press.

Mitrani, V. B., De Santis, J. P., McCabe, B. E., Deleon, D. A., Gattamorta, K. A., & Leblanc, N. M. (2017). The impact of parental reaction to sexual orientation on depressive symptoms and sexual risk behavior among Hispanic men who have sex with men. *Archives of Psychiatric Nursing*, *31*(4), 352–358. https://doi.org/10.1016/j.apnu.2017.04.004

Nadel, L., Hupbach, A., Hardt, O., & Gomez, R. (2008). Episodic memory: Reconsolidation. In E. Dere, A. Easton, L. Nadel, & J. P. Huston (Eds.), *Handbook of behavioral neuroscience* (Vol. 18, pp. 43–56). Elsevier. https://doi.org/10.1016/S1569-7339(08)00204-X

Needham, B. L., & Austin, E. L. (2010). Sexual orientation, parental support, and health during the transition to young adulthood. *Journal of Youth and Adolescence*, *39*(10), 1189–1198. https://doi.org/10.1007/s10964-010-9533-6

Nichols, M. P., & Colapinto, J. (2017). Enactment in structural family therapy. In J. Lebow, A. Chambers, & D. C. Breunlin (Eds.), *Encyclopedia of couple and family therapy* (pp. 1–4). Springer International Publishing.

Norwood, K. (2012). Transitioning meanings? Family members' communicative struggles surrounding transgender identity. *Journal of Family Communication*, *12*(1), 75–92. https://doi.org/10.1080/15267431.2010.509283

Pachankis, J. E., Goldfried, M. R., & Ramrattan, M. E. (2008). Extension of the rejection sensitivity construct to the interpersonal functioning of gay men. *Journal of Consulting and Clinical Psychology*, *76*(2), 306–317. https://doi.org/10.1037/0022-006X.76.2.306

Pachankis, J. E., Sullivan, T. J., & Moore, N. F. (2018). A 7-year longitudinal study of sexual minority young men's parental relationships and mental health.

Journal of Family Psychology, 32(8), 1068–1077. https://doi.org/10.1037/fam0000427

Padilla, Y. C., Crisp, C., & Rew, D. L. (2010). Parental acceptance and illegal drug use among gay, lesbian, and bisexual adolescents: Results from a national survey. *Social Work, 55*(3), 265–275. https://doi.org/10.1093/sw/55.3.265

Parra, L. A., Bell, T. S., Benibgui, M., Helm, J. L., & Hastings, P. D. (2018). The buffering effect of peer support on the links between family rejection and psychosocial adjustment in LGB emerging adults. *Journal of Social and Personal Relationships, 35*(6), 854–871. https://doi.org/10.1177/0265407517699713 (Corrigendum published July 31, 2017, *Journal of Social and Personal Relationships, 34*[7], 1145. https://doi.org/10.1177/0265407517725426)

Pascual-Leone, A., & Greenberg, L. S. (2007). Emotional processing in experiential therapy: Why "the only way out is through." *Journal of Consulting and Clinical Psychology, 75*(6), 875–887. https://doi.org/10.1037/0022-006X.75.6.875

Pascual-Leone, A., & Kramer, U. (2019). How clients "change emotion with emotion": Sequences in emotional processing and their clinical implications. In L. S. Greenberg & R. N. Goldman (Eds.), *Clinical handbook of emotion-focused therapy* (pp. 147–170). American Psychological Association. https://doi.org/10.1037/0000112-007

PBS News Weekend. (2015, August 2). *Israeli teen stabbed at Gay Pride parade dies*. PBS. https://www.pbs.org/newshour/world/israeli-teen-stabbed-gay-pride-parade-dies

Pearlman, S. F. (2006). Terms of connection: Mother-talk about female-to-male transgender children. *Journal of GLBT Family Studies, 2*(3–4), 93–122. https://doi.org/10.1300/J461v02n03_06

Poushter, J., & Kent, N. (2020, June 25). *The global divide on homosexuality persists* (Report). Pew Research Center. https://www.pewresearch.org/global/2020/06/25/global-divide-on-homosexuality-persists/

Remafedi, G., Farrow, J. A., & Deisher, R. W. (1991). Risk factors for attempted suicide in gay and bisexual youth. *Pediatrics, 87*(6), 869–875. https://doi.org/10.1542/peds.87.6.869

Reynolds, W. M., & Mazza, J. J. (1999). Assessment of suicidal ideation in inner-city children and young adolescents: Reliability and validity of the Suicidal Ideation Questionnaire-JR. *School Psychology Review, 28*(1), 17–30. https://doi.org/10.1080/02796015.1999.12085945

Rochman, D., Diamond, G. M., & Amir, O. (2008). Unresolved anger and sadness: Identifying vocal acoustical correlates. *Journal of Counseling Psychology, 55*(4), 505–517. https://doi.org/10.1037/a0013720

Rohrbaugh, M. J. (2014). Old wine in new bottles: Decanting systemic family process research in the era of evidence-based practice. *Family Process, 53*(3), 434–444. https://doi.org/10.1111/famp.12079

Rosenkrantz, D. E., Rostosky, S. S., Toland, M. D., & Dueber, D. M. (2020). Cognitive–affective and religious values associated with parental acceptance of an LGBT child. *Psychology of Sexual Orientation and Gender Diversity, 7*(1), 55–65. https://doi.org/10.1037/sgd0000355

Rothman, E. F., Sullivan, M., Keyes, S., & Boehmer, U. (2012). Parents' supportive reactions to sexual orientation disclosure associated with better health: Results from a population-based survey of LGB adults in Massachusetts. *Journal of Homosexuality, 59*(2), 186–200. https://doi.org/10.1080/00918369.2012.648878

Russon, J., Morrissey, J., Dellinger, J., Jin, B., & Diamond, G. (2021). Implementing attachment-based family therapy for depressed and suicidal adolescents and young adults in LGBTQ+ services: Feasibility, acceptability, and preliminary effectiveness. *Crisis.* Advance online publication. https://doi.org/10.1027/0227-5910/a000821

Ryan, C., Huebner, D., Diaz, R. M., & Sanchez, J. (2009). Family rejection as a predictor of negative health outcomes in White and Latino lesbian, gay, and bisexual young adults. *Pediatrics, 123*(1), 346–352. https://doi.org/10.1542/peds.2007-3524

Ryan, C., Russell, S. T., Huebner, D., Diaz, R., & Sanchez, J. (2010). Family acceptance in adolescence and the health of LGBT young adults. *Journal of Child and Adolescent Psychiatric Nursing, 23*(4), 205–213. https://doi.org/10.1111/j.1744-6171.2010.00246.x

Safran, J. D., & Greenberg, L. S. (1991). *Emotion, psychotherapy, and change.* Guilford Press.

Salerno, J. P., Gattamorta, K. A., & Williams, N. D. (2022). Impact of family rejection and racism on sexual and gender minority stress among LGBTQ young people of color during COVID-19. *Psychological Trauma: Theory, Research, Practice, and Policy.* Advance online publication. https://doi.org/10.1037/tra0001254

Saltzburg, S. (2004). Learning that an adolescent child is gay or lesbian: The parent experience. *Social Work, 49*(1), 109–118. https://doi.org/10.1093/sw/49.1.109

Samarova, V., Shilo, G., & Diamond, G. M. (2014). Changes in youths' perceived parental acceptance of their sexual minority status over time. *Journal of Research on Adolescence, 24*(4), 681–688. https://doi.org/10.1111/jora.12071

Savin-Williams, R. C. (1989). Parental influences on the self-esteem of gay and lesbian youths: A reflected appraisals model. *Journal of Homosexuality, 17*(1–2), 93–110. https://doi.org/10.1300/J082v17n01_04

Savin-Williams, R. C. (2001). *Mom, Dad. I'm gay. How families negotiate coming out.* American Psychological Association. https://doi.org/10.1037/10437-000

Shao, J., Chang, E. S., & Chen, C. (2018). The relative importance of parent–child dynamics and minority stress on the psychological adjustment of LGBs in China. *Journal of Counseling Psychology, 65*(5), 598–604. https://doi.org/10.1037/cou0000281

Sheets, R. L., Jr., & Mohr, J. J. (2009). Perceived social support from friends and family and psychosocial functioning in bisexual young adult college students.

Journal of Counseling Psychology, 56(1), 152–163. https://doi.org/10.1037/0022-0167.56.1.152

Shelef, K., Diamond, G. M., Diamond, G. S., & Liddle, H. A. (2005). Adolescent and parent alliance and treatment outcome in multidimensional family therapy. *Journal of Consulting and Clinical Psychology, 73*(4), 689–698. https://doi.org/10.1037/0022-006X.73.4.689

Shilo, G., Antebi, N., & Mor, Z. (2015). Individual and community resilience factors among lesbian, gay, bisexual, queer and questioning youth and adults in Israel. *American Journal of Community Psychology, 55*(1–2), 215–227. https://doi.org/10.1007/s10464-014-9693-8

Shilo, G., & Savaya, R. (2011). Effects of family and friend support on LGB youths' mental health and sexual orientation milestones. *Family Relations, 60*(3), 318–330. https://doi.org/10.1111/j.1741-3729.2011.00648.x

Shpigel, M. S., & Diamond, G. M. (2014). Good versus poor therapeutic alliances with non-accepting parents of same-sex oriented adolescents and young adults: A qualitative study. *Psychotherapy Research, 24*(3), 376–391. https://doi.org/10.1080/10503307.2013.856043

Simons, L., Schrager, S. M., Clark, L. F., Belzer, M., & Olson, J. (2013). Parental support and mental health among transgender adolescents. *The Journal of Adolescent Health, 53*(6), 791–793. https://doi.org/10.1016/j.jadohealth.2013.07.019

Snapp, S. D., Watson, R. J., Russell, S. T., Diaz, R. M., & Ryan, C. (2015). Social support networks for LGBT young adults: Low cost strategies for positive adjustment. *Family Relations, 64*(3), 420–430. https://doi.org/10.1111/fare.12124

Stone Fish, L., & Harvey, R. G. (2005). *Nurturing queer youth: Family therapy transformed.* Norton Professional Books.

Strifler, Y., Zisenwine, T., & Diamond, G. M. (2022). Parents' reflective functioning and their agreement on treatment goals in attachment-based family therapy for sexual and gender minority young adults and their nonaccepting parents. *Journal of Marital and Family Therapy.* Advance online publication. https://doi.org/10.1111/jmft.12581

Sue, D. W. (2010). *Microaggressions and marginality: Manifestation, dynamics, and impact.* John Wiley & Sons.

Tate, D. P., & Patterson, C. J. (2019). Sexual orientation, relationships with parents, stress, and depressive symptoms among adults. *Journal of GLBT Family Studies, 15*(3), 256–271. https://doi.org/10.1080/1550428X.2018.1486263

The Times of Israel Staff. (2022, May 18). Pride march in Netivot nixed after bullet sent to organizer's mother. *The Times of Israel.* https://www.timesofisrael.com/pride-march-in-netivot-nixed-after-bullet-sent-to-organizers-mother/

Trinke, S. J., & Bartholomew, K. (1997). Hierarchies of attachment relationships in young adulthood. *Journal of Social and Personal Relationships, 14*(5), 603–625. https://doi.org/10.1177/0265407597145002

Tsvieli, N., & Diamond, G. M. (2018). Therapist interventions and emotional processing in attachment-based family therapy for unresolved anger. *Psychotherapy*, *55*(3), 289–297. https://doi.org/10.1037/pst0000158

Tsvieli, N., Lifshitz, C., & Diamond, G. M. (2022). Corrective attachment episodes in attachment-based family therapy: The power of enactment. *Psychotherapy Research*, *32*(2), 209–222. https://doi.org/10.1080/10503307.2021.1913295

Tsvieli, N., Nir-Gottlieb, O., Lifshitz, C., Diamond, G. S., Kobak, R., & Diamond, G. M. (2020). Therapist interventions associated with productive emotional processing in the context of attachment-based family therapy for depressed and suicidal adolescents. *Family Process*, *59*(2), 428–444. https://doi.org/10.1111/famp.12445

van der Toorn, J., Jost, J. T., Packer, D. J., Noorbaloochi, S., & Van Bavel, J. J. (2017). In defense of tradition: Religiosity, conservatism, and opposition to same-sex marriage in North America. *Personality and Social Psychology Bulletin*, *43*(10), 1455–1468. https://doi.org/10.1177/0146167217718523

van Wel, F., Linssen, H., & Abma, R. (2000). The parental bond and the well-being of adolescents and young adults. *Journal of Youth and Adolescence*, *29*(3), 307–318. https://doi.org/10.1023/A:1005195624757

van Wel, F., ter Bogt, T., & Raaijmakers, Q. (2002). Changes in the parental bond and the well-being of adolescents and young adults. *Adolescence*, *37*(146), 317–333.

Wahlig, J. L. (2015). Losing the child they thought they had: Therapeutic suggestions for an ambiguous loss perspective with parents of a transgender child. *Journal of GLBT Family Studies*, *11*(4), 305–326. https://doi.org/10.1080/1550428X.2014.945676

Zuccarini, D., Johnson, S. M., Dalgleish, T. L., & Makinen, J. A. (2013). Forgiveness and reconciliation in emotionally focused therapy for couples: The client change process and therapist interventions. *Journal of Marital and Family Therapy*, *39*(2), 148–162. https://doi.org/10.1111/j.1752-0606.2012.00287.x

Index

About the Authors

Gary M. Diamond, PhD, is a professor in the Department of Psychology at Ben-Gurion University in Israel. He is a licensed clinical psychologist and family therapist as well as the director and chief psychologist at the Ben-Gurion University Community Clinic. One of the primary developers of attachment-based family therapy (ABFT), in 2014 he coauthored with Guy S. Diamond (no family relation) and Suzanne A. Levy the book *Attachment-Based Family Therapy for Depressed Adolescents*, published by the American Psychological Association. He also took the lead in adapting ABFT for use with lesbian, gay, and bisexual depressed and suicidal adolescents and, more recently, extended this work to sexual and gender minority young adults and their nonaccepting parents.

Dr. Diamond's research examines the processes and outcomes of ABFT. He has studied the therapeutic alliance in family therapy, emotional processing, attachment anxiety and avoidance, parental responsiveness and parental acceptance, and corrective attachment episodes. In 2014, along with Guy S. Diamond, he received the American Foundation for Suicide Prevention's annual research award. He trains people internationally in ABFT for sexual and gender minority adolescents and young adults. You are invited to visit https://www.bgupsychotherapyresearch.org/ to read more about his work.

Rotem Boruchovitz-Zamir, MA, is a doctoral student and clinical psychology intern at Ben-Gurion University in Israel. She collaborated in adapting attachment-based family therapy for sexual and gender minority young adults and their nonaccepting parents (ABFT-SGM). She is also an expert ABFT-SGM therapist and served as a therapist on the first ABFT-SGM clinical trial. Her dissertation research examined how changes in parental behavior over the course of ABFT-SGM were associated with young adults' sense of parental acceptance and rejection.